The Word of Wisdom

Hope, Healing, and the Destroying Angel

Cassidy and Jordan Gundersen

EDITED BY:

Judy Shepherd and Nicole Reeder

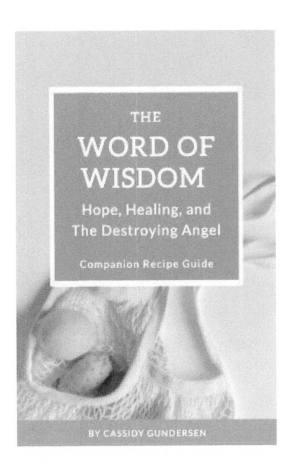

THE

WORD OF WISDOM

Hope, Healing, and The Destroying Angel

Companion Recipe Guide

BY CASSIDY GUNDERSEN

Get the FREE Companion Recipe Guide

Go to wordofwisdombook.com/recipes

Foreword

2020. What a time we live in: a time of fear, a time of anger, a time of division, a time of confusion, a time of mistrust, and a perfect time for Cassidy and Jordan to release *The Word of Wisdom: Hope Healing and the Destroying Angel.*

It reminds me of another desperate time when the brother of my third-great-grandfather, Hyrum Smith, was concerned about the similar turmoil in his day. His brother Joseph asked the Lord what was true, and many truths were revealed through this latter-day prophet. One of these revealed truths is the Word of Wisdom (Doctrine and Covenants Section 89) recorded verbatim from the mouth of the Lord.

I was raised in a family with "goodly parents" who, with temperance, adhered to these revealed truths. Later in life as I lectured internationally, people thought I was brilliant when I explained health principles that were instilled in me from my family. But these principles came from the Word of Wisdom as revealed from God.

While all other institutes of higher learning constantly change teachings of health and diet, our School of Natural Healing has never changed its curriculum on diet because it was based on revealed truth contained in the 89th Section of the Doctrine and Covenants.

Cassidy and Jordan cut through all the confusion on health in their excellent new book which clarifies the truths contained in the Word of Wisdom (D&C 89). Their excellent treatise annotates all references from authorities, health professionals, and scientific studies.

The simple truths contained in the Word of Wisdom, if followed with temperance, will bless us with health in our navel (good digestion) and marrow in our bones (a strong immune system). This will protect us from all invaders including viruses from cows, pigs, birds, bats, or from Mars. We are all also promised, from God, that if we live this whole commandment "the destroying angel will pass us by as the children of Israel and not slay us." In our day, we need not fear pandemics. Instead of putting lambs' blood on our door frames, as the Israelites of old, we can avoid them by adhering to our health code, the Word of Wisdom.

I believe all households can be saved temporally today by adhering to these truths taught in the 89th Section and clarified in Cassidy and Jordan Gundersen's new release *The Word of Wisdom: Hope, Healing, and the Destroying Angel.*

David W. Christopher, MH
Director, School of Natural Healing

Introduction

When we initially set out to write this book, we were hoping to create something like a pamphlet to discuss our experience with the principles in the Word of Wisdom using supporting quotes from many prophets of this dispensation. However, as we began, it became clear that we couldn't confine all of what we learned to a pamphlet. Additionally, the deeper we went into the Word of Wisdom, the more we realized how much the scriptures in general talk about what to do to keep our bodies healthy.

This book is the culmination of our efforts to understand what the Lord has said about health in the scriptures. We focus on what has been revealed in these last days, namely the Word of Wisdom, by discussing the history of the Word of Wisdom, and then reviewing the revelation chronologically, discussing each of the principles contained therein. For ease, we have broken the dietary principles into three categories, the 'Don'ts', the 'Sometimes', and the 'Dos.' A whole chapter is devoted to the use of herbs in the Lord's pattern of healing. Finally, we will discuss the role the Word of Wisdom will play regarding the destroying angel in the last days. Through all of this, we will often refer to Noah Webster's 1828 version of An American Dictionary of the English Language. This is because language changes over time, and the meanings of words often change as well. By referring to this dictionary, commonly regarded as the authority on biblical words and early 19th century America, we can often gain a clearer understanding of what the Lord was trying to convey in certain passages and what the Saints of the day understood them to mean. Throughout the book, the default speaker is both of us, unless otherwise specified. For instance, we will write something like "I (Cassidy)" to clarify when only one of us is speaking.

Certainly, we do not understand everything about health or the scriptures. However, we have lived the principles that will be discussed in this book and have seen great blessings for doing so. We have also helped many other people find greater health as they live these principles through our nutrition-based business, Spiro Health & Wellness.

We feel that this book is so important for Church members in these last days largely because much of the information you will read has been lost or forgotten, leading to poor health outcomes for many in the Church. We are quite certain that some of the things you will read may shock you—specifically, what many of the prophets (and the scriptures) have said regarding the Word of Wisdom and other health practices. While we were shocked when we read them as well, what many scriptures and prophets have declared in days past is now being confirmed by modern research. We keep a discussion of academic research and science to a minimum while pointing out instances where science has confirmed what has already been revealed. Here we would like to remind the reader that the Word of Wisdom is a religious belief, not a scientific one. Scholarly corroboration can now be found for many of the principles in the revelation. However, our religious convictions and testimony should be forged through faith, intense study, prayer, and personal experience. All truth comes from God, and as such, we ought to rely on His Word and not man's. We would be building a foundation upon sand if we relied on data, science, and studies to mold our religious beliefs. Science is ever changing, but the decrees of God are eternal. With all of this in mind, we will assume that the reader already has a basic understanding and testimony of the Word of Wisdom as we discuss modern research that supports the principles in this God-given code of health.

We don't profess to have all the answers, nor do we claim authority to speak for the Church of Jesus Christ of Latter-day Saints. We should point out that the Church has stated on multiple occasions, "Not every statement made by a Church leader, past or present, necessarily constitutes doctrine. A single statement made by a single leader on a single occasion often represents a personal, though well-considered, opinion, but is not meant to be officially binding for the whole Church."[1] The doctrines of the Church are to be found in the scriptures; are consistently taught by the Brethren over time, and can be confirmed by the Holy Ghost. On this matter, Joseph Fielding Smith succinctly explained:

> "It makes no difference what is written or what anyone has said, if what has been said is in conflict with what the Lord has revealed, we can set it aside. **My words, and the teaching of any other member of the Church, high or low, if they do not square with the revelations, we need not accept them.** Let us have this matter clear. We have accepted the four standard works as the measuring yardsticks, or balances, by which we measure every man's doctrine."[2]

Therefore, if something we state in this book does not meet this standard, you can cast it aside as not constituting doctrine. However, that does not necessarily mean it is not a true principle. This book was not written to tell you what you should think about the Word of Wisdom or to criticize *any* other member's health practices, beliefs, or commitment to God and the Word of Wisdom. Rather, it is to highlight material that enhances an understanding of the principles contained in the scriptures. Read with an open mind, then search it out and study it for yourself. Our invitation is similar to what Jesus taught His disciples in the New Testament: "If any man will do his will, he shall know of the doctrine, whether it be of God, or whether I speak of myself."[3] Experience is one of the ultimate teachers. Experiment on the word, and see if it is good.

---

[1] "Approaching Mormon Doctrine," Church of Jesus Christ of Latter-day Saints Newsroom, Salt Lake City, 4 May 2007.
[2] Joseph Fielding Smith, *Doctrines of Salvation*, edited by Bruce R. McConkie, vol. 3, (Salt Lake City, UT: Bookcraft, 1956), p. 203.
[3] John 7:17.

Our lives have been forever changed by the information found in this book. It is our hope that our experience and the information we share can help change your life for the better as well.

Chapter One

Why You Need the Word of Wisdom

"I, the Lord, am bound when ye do
what I say; but when ye do not what I
say, ye have no promise."
Doctrine & Covenants 82:10

I (Cassidy) never did anything half-hearted. I was involved in every club, activity, or competition that existed in small town Ammon, Idaho. I enjoyed being the center of attention, which often landed me center stage in pageants, plays, and the debate team. I excelled in each of these activities, which put a great deal of stress on my young body. When I was only 13, I embarked on a long, challenging road of health problems with the onset of what would become chronic kidney stones. The first time I had one I remember thinking I was going to die. I was in so much pain! I couldn't do anything but lay on the ground in a fetal position throwing up, sometimes for over 24 hours. I experienced these kidney stones on and off every few months from that point forward.

I thought that was the extent of my health woes, but as I grew older it seemed like my body was beginning to fall apart. By the time I was 20, I was crowned as Miss Idaho, was an award-winning member of the Model United Nations team at BYU, and was also a contestant on the popular tv show, "American Idol." The amount of stress in my life began to feel like more than I could bear, and my body started to give up. Before long, I was plagued with debilitating PMS symptoms, chronic fatigue, migraines, and digestive problems. Some are shocked to learn that I only had a bowel movement once or twice every month. But I didn't know any different, so I didn't see it as a problem. I assumed bowel movements were painful and bloody for everyone, just as they were for me.

In 2012, I received my mission call to serve in the Canada, Winnipeg mission. When I submitted my papers, I asked God to send me to the hardest mission in the world (which is a story for another book). Suffice it to say, the Lord answered my prayers. While serving in the frigid north, my health took a turn for the worse; I gained 60 lbs. rapidly, I started experiencing extreme adrenal fatigue, and my migraines worsened.

One morning, while on a run with my companion, half of my body went numb. I wasn't sure what to do, so they rushed me to the hospital. I waited in the ER room for an entire day before meeting with a doctor. He ran a series of tests, including an MRI, with no diagnoses.

Throughout my mission, my condition worsened to the point that I was experiencing severe stomach cramps and pain when having a bowel movement. I started to find a significant amount of blood in my stool and finally decided I needed to go to the doctor again. After more tests than I can count, I was diagnosed with Crohn's Disease. I was both terrified and relieved to finally have a diagnosis. That night, I went back to my apartment and just cried. I was so frustrated! Here I was, dedicating my entire life to the Lord and trying to teach as many people as possible, and my body was giving out. I couldn't make it through an entire day of teaching. I was constantly exhausted and in pain. Why wasn't the Lord stepping in to heal my ailments when I was trying to do His work?

Amidst all of this, one night I turned to my patriarchal blessing. I began reading and saw an entire section dedicated to the blessings I would have from obeying the Word of Wisdom.

Reading this made me even angrier. I was promised health and strength as I lived the Word of Wisdom—neither of which I had at the time. I had never drunk coffee or alcohol. I had never smoked a cigarette or had tea. "I have kept the Word of Wisdom perfectly my entire life, and yet I have no blessings," was the thought running through my mind. Reading these promises and feeling like they could not be realized no matter how obedient I was to the commandment was more than I could bear. I put away my patriarchal blessing and cried myself to sleep.

When I returned home, I began meeting with an increasing number of doctors and specialists to understand more about my health problems. More doctors, more tests, more procedures, and nothing seemed to change. In desperation, I asked my gastroenterologist during one appointment which foods I should eat and which I should avoid. He assured me food didn't impact my digestion and that I just needed to keep taking the medications prescribed to me. Something about that didn't resonate well with me. I knew very little about nutrition at the time, but I was fairly sure that food choices impacted digestion. Either way, I knew there had to be another path other than medicating myself into numbness.

In 2015, I met and married my husband, Jordan. He was supportive and loving with me as I faced many difficult days, sometimes staying in bed all day. Several months after our marriage, I was diagnosed with 12 different health conditions, including pre-lupus, pre-diabetes, tendonitis, adrenal fatigue, and more. At one particularly difficult visit, the doctor informed my husband and me that given the condition of my body, I would likely die young. Struggling to swallow the implications of these diagnoses himself, Jordan assured me that we would find a way to get me better. He chose to not accept this as the dead-end it seemed to be. At this same appointment, however, we discovered that Jordan, who we always thought was very healthy, had early warning signs of heart disease. Here he was, a skinny 23-year-old, who had a steadily increasing risk of a heart attack!

That day was a turning point. This was when I knew that we had to take our health into our own hands. We began trying to eat healthier, and I tried to learn as much as I could about nutrition. We visited a functional medicine doctor who supported dietary intervention, and I was sure this would be our answer. We were quickly put on a 'keto diet,' and I began eating cleaner than I ever had before. Though my energy began to increase, I was still facing most of the same issues, just with marginally less severity.

It was during this period that I convinced my husband to go to a clean eating restaurant I had just heard about in Springville, Utah called Ginger's Garden Cafe. We went for lunch, and next to our table was a small book titled *Just What is the Word of Wisdom*. In it, Dr. John Christopher, a world-renowned herbalist, argued that the dietary principles of the Word of Wisdom were a lot more than just avoiding coffee, tea, tobacco, alcohol, and drugs. For example, did you know that the Word of Wisdom tells us exactly what kinds of foods we should eat? Did you know that the Word of Wisdom tells us to spare God's creatures? Even more, did you also know that an overwhelming majority of modern prophets have echoed the same sentiments concerning the Word of Wisdom? Later in this book, we will present some of this evidence we have found about each of these topics. It is our belief that many of these principles are necessary in order to obtain *all* of the blessings of the Word of Wisdom.

This was the first time in my life it had ever occurred to me that perhaps my daily meat consumption was not in harmony with the principles in the Word of Wisdom. Additionally, I had been avoiding fruits and grains like the plague on our new diet. Yet the Word of Wisdom advocated generous use of these as well. I was completely shocked!

My husband and I spent the next week studying every talk, article, book, podcast, and YouTube video we could find on the Word of Wisdom. It was like a whole new world was opened to us, and we wanted to learn all we could. The more I read, the more I realized I was living far beneath my privileges when it came to the Word of Wisdom. It was no wonder my body was plagued with so many ailments. My Maker had designed a beautiful health plan for me, and I had simply ignored a great majority of it, thinking that I had been following it, for over 24 years!

I decided it was time to step forward in faith, even though it was against everything I had been learning from my doctor and others. I decided to follow *all* of the Lord's instructions in the Word of Wisdom and to specifically focus on fruits, vegetables, grains, and other herbs. I began immediately, and Jordan, who was a little more hesitant initially, agreed to a 2-week trial of this lifestyle. Within days, we felt better than we ever had before! I was amazed at just how great I felt eating exactly as the Lord had advised. These feelings only increased, and I knew that we could never go back to the way things were before.

As time went on, we began to live the Word of Wisdom with more and more exactness. I discovered dozens of fruits and vegetables I had never heard of before and excitedly began adding them to our diet. After six months, I returned to the doctor to do more tests and bloodwork. They were astonished to discover that the results came back completely clean for the first time in my life. I was healed! Truly, this is a miracle, given just how poor the condition of my body had been. I went from near my death bed, to the healthiest of my life all thanks to the Lord. I can do things now with ease that I never thought my body could handle. If it weren't for the Word of Wisdom, I'm not sure I would even be alive today. And with what we would later discover, the Word of Wisdom will play a critical role in events of the last days.

The Current State of Health in the Church

If you're reading this book, you may have had similar thoughts as I did: "I'm living the Word of Wisdom, so why am I not receiving the promised blessings?" We (Cassidy and Jordan) are certain that many members of the Church have had this question at some point or another. It was hard for us to fathom just how unhealthy many Church members are.

A recent study from Brigham Young University showed that Church members were 34% more likely to be obese than members of other religions.[1] Additionally, over 70% of Latter-day Saint adults 35 years and older are overweight.[2] In youth, nearly 45% are overweight.[3] Many of these numbers are either on par with those of the rest of the world or worse. It would appear that, despite having a code of health, the outcomes are pretty much the same as those that don't adhere to one. So what is the deal?

The Promises of the Word of Wisdom

One of the most frustrating things for Cassidy was being promised the blessings of the Word of Wisdom, not only in the scriptures, but also in her patriarchal blessing if she obeyed. The blessings promised in Section 89 related to health are that the doers "shall receive health in their navel and marrow to their bones" and that they "shall run and not be weary, and shall walk and not faint."[4] The Lord even promises that the one who obeys "shall find wisdom and great treasures of knowledge, even hidden treasures."[5] The Lord promises that if we obey, He will even reveal to us the mysteries of His kingdom as He revealed to Nephi as a young boy! How incredible is that?

---

[1] Grant Grayson, "The Mormon Obesity Epidemic: Why Diet Soft Drinks Make Us Fat," LDS Living, 7 June 2017.
[2] Ibid.
[3] Ibid.
[4] Doctrine and Covenants 89:18, 20.
[5] Doctrine and Covenants 89:19.

Of the importance of these spiritual treasures, President Spencer W. Kimball said the following:

"What could be so priceless as wisdom and knowledge, even hidden treasures? Surely the treasures here referred to are not those of scientific accomplishments. Such will come revealed as light from heaven discovered through the research of men, but these hidden treasures of knowledge in the revelation are those which can be had only by use of the keys given which are: 'Walking in obedience.' And while the discoveries in the physical world are very important to us here in mortality, the spiritual discovery of a knowledge of God and his program reach into and through eternity."[6]

The Word of Wisdom is so important because our body and our spirit are connected. When our body suffers, our spirit suffers as well. One of the main objectives of our existence as spiritual beings is to learn how to have a physical experience and subdue our body to the will of our spirit. By living the Word of Wisdom, we place our body in a state to receive in great measure the knowledge of God to achieve that end and become like God.

One of the greatest things about God is that He does not promise blessings which He does not intend to give. He is a compassionate and consistent God. He tells us that He is "bound" to bless us when we do what He says. In other words, if we are following the principles that are prerequisites for the blessings, He has no choice but to bless us. By His own law and standard, we have claim upon the blessings when we follow His commands. This has to be one of the most enlightening and enabling aspects of the Restored Gospel!

Now, this doesn't mean that we'll never experience anything hard in our lives, because part of our existence is to pass through

---

[6] Spencer W. Kimball, *Conference Report*, October 1944, p. 42.

trials. In regards to the Word of Wisdom, then Elder Gordon B. Hinckley taught:

> "I am not saying that disease will not come, that death will not strike. Death is a part of the divine plan, a necessary step in the eternal life of the sons and daughters of God. But I do not hesitate to say that in this brief but inclusive statement of the Lord is found counsel, given with a promise, which, if more widely observed, would save untold pain and suffering and lead not only to increased physical well-being but also to great and satisfying 'treasures of knowledge' of the things of God."[7]

Indeed, if we were to observe these principles better, we might be able to realize the Lord's promises more abundantly–those of health, strength, energy, and increased spirituality.

How To Read the Word of Wisdom

A common sentiment that we often hear is, "I don't partake of any of the forbidden substances in the Word of Wisdom, but I'm still sick!" We are sympathetic to this plight because it was once our own. However, if we feel that we're not receiving the promised blessings, shouldn't we then look at the Word of Wisdom from a different perspective? This different perspective we speak of is not anything new. Rather it is one that seems to have been lost in the Church over the last several decades but was once taught consistently and frequently beginning with the Prophet Joseph Smith. While some perceived health experts in the Church believe that there is nothing to be gained from a strict or literal interpretation of the Word of Wisdom, the voice of many latter-day prophets have taught otherwise.[8] As Joseph Smith himself recorded, the unanimous consent of the High Council declared, "we will not fellowship any ordained member

---

[7] Gordon B. Hinckley, "Come and Partake," *Ensign*, May 1986, p. 49.
[8] Benjamin Bikman, "The Plagues of Prosperity," BYU Forum Address, 17 July 2018.

who will not, or does not observe the Word of Wisdom **according to its literal meaning.**"[9] In other words, the revelation we know as Section 89 means what it says.

Unfortunately, many members of the Church believe that the Word of Wisdom is up for interpretation by each member. Of course, there may be some room for interpretation in certain circumstances; however, as Joseph Fielding Smith said, "The word of Wisdom is a basic law. It points the way and gives us ample instruction in regard to both food and drink, good for the body and also detrimental. If we sincerely follow what is written with the aid of the Spirit of the Lord, we need no further counsel."[10] Rather than decide for ourselves what the revelation means, maybe we should try to understand what God meant by it and how we can conform to its principles. In a similar vein, President Heber J. Grant taught the need to follow all of the Lord's requirements. In 1931 he said:

> "I have met any number of people who have said the Word of Wisdom is not a command from the Lord, that it is not given by way of commandment. But the Word of Wisdom is the will of the Lord and the Lord says in the words that I have just read that it is not meet that we should be commanded in all things. . . One of the best ways in all the world to bring to pass much righteousness is to set an example as a conscientious, God-fearing Latter-day Saint, **observing all of the requirements of the Lord.**"[11]

Indeed, we are not commanded in all things. Section 89 declares that the Word of Wisdom was given as a "principle with promise, adapted to the capacity of the weak and the weakest of

---

[9] History of the Church, vol. 2, p. 482, general meeting of the Church 28 May 1837, emphasis added.
[10] Joseph Fielding Smith, *Answers to Gospel Questions*, vol. 1, (Salt Lake City, UT: Deseret Book Company, 1957), p. 199.
[11] Heber J. Grant, *Conference Report*, April 1931, pp. 12-13, emphasis added.

all saints, who are or can be called saints." If this code of health is a set of principles adapted for the *weakest* of Saints, could this be a lower law, and is there a higher law? We won't speculate on the implications or possible meaning here but will leave that for the private consideration and pondering of the reader. The purpose of this book could be summarized well by the words of Elder Boyd K. Packer: "While the Word of Wisdom requires strict obedience, in return it promises health, great treasures of knowledge, and that redemption bought for us by the Lamb of God, who was slain that we might be redeemed."

The answer to many of today's challenges and many of the challenges in the future can be found in the Word of Wisdom. We don't have anything new to present to you in this book than what can already be found in the scriptures and the words of the prophets; we have merely organized them in what we feel is an interesting and digestible manner. Sure, we may add modern research that enables us to see the principles practically. But the principles in the Word of Wisdom are self-evident. Live them and you will see. Greater health and spiritual strength *can* be found today, and the Lord's promise of protection in the last days *can* be realized.

Chapter Two

History of the Word of Wisdom

"And the voice of warning shall be unto all
people, by the mouths of my disciples, whom
I have chosen in these last days."
Doctrine and Covenants 1:4

The revelation in Doctrine and Covenants Section 89, more commonly known as the "Word of Wisdom," was received by Joseph Smith in 1833 in Kirtland, Ohio. It is officially accepted as scripture by the Church of Jesus Christ of Latter-Day Saints, and an understanding of it is currently a prerequisite to hold a temple recommend. The Word of Wisdom has a long history–a history more nuanced than most members of the Church realize. With an understanding of the context of the revelation, the time in which it was given, and the history of it since, we can begin to grasp why it should be more important in our lives.

A Lack of Temperance

In the mid 1800s, tobacco, alcohol, tea, and coffee were regularly consumed by most members of society, much like they are today. Tobacco was still used frequently in various forms by the medical world, as it was thought to cure many ailments.[1] Beyond its medicinal purposes, it was routinely used for enjoyment via smoking and chewing.

---

[1] Anne Charlton, "Medicinal uses of tobacco in history," *Journal of the Royal Society of Medicine*, June 2004.

Alcohol was also in great demand. In fact, during this time, Americans consumed more alcohol than at any other time before or since. The average person drank seven and a half gallons of pure alcohol a year in the 1800s.[2] Today, the average American drinks around two gallons each year.[3] One author referred to America during this time as the "alcoholic republic," saying, "Americans drank at home and abroad, alone and together, at work and at play. Americans drank before meals, with meals and after meals. They drank while working in the fields and while traveling across half a continent."[4] Coffee and Tea were no exception, as they were consumed in large quantities by men, women, and children alike. One prominent Church historian writes, "By the time Joseph Smith moved to Kirtland, Ohio, in 1831, more Americans were beginning to become concerned with social vices generally and alcohol abuse especially. Besides slavery, gambling, and political corruption, debate swirled about the appropriate use of alcohol. Reformers advocated temperance or the moderate use of alcohol."[5]

While alcohol and other similar beverages were extremely popular, there was a growing temperance movement taking shape around the same time. Joseph Smith was not the first or only voice to speak against alcohol and other excitotoxins.[6] Starting in 1805, the temperance movement quickly gained popularity across the country. However, just because the temperance movement happened during the time in which the Word of Wisdom was revealed does not necessarily mean that it was a product of the movement itself. Joseph may have admired

---

[2] Jane O'Brien, "The Time When Americans Drank All Day Long", *BBC News*, March 2015.

[3] Alice Felt Tyler, *Freedom's Ferment*, (New York: Harper and Row, 1944) p. 312.

[4] W. J. Rorabaugh, *The Alcoholic Republic: An American Tradition*, (New York: Oxford University Press, 1979), pp. 20-21.

[5] Steven C. Harper, *Setting the Record Straight: The Word of Wisdom*, (Orem, UT: Millennial Press, 2007), p. 28.

[6] Sylvester E Graham, *The Aesculapian Tablets of the Nineteenth Century* (Providence Weeden and Cory,1834) p vii.

or been sympathetic to some of the temperance principles, but we do not have any recorded statements from him about his feelings on the matter. Therefore, we choose not to make such a conclusion as to the relationship of the temperance movement to the Word of Wisdom.

Early American Diet and Health

During the 1800s, the standard American diet consisted primarily of locally grown fruits, vegetables, beans, and grains. Most were farmers, and that was sufficient to sustain their family's needs, occasionally trading with community members to supplement what they didn't grow themselves. Since railroads were not yet well established, importing other foods was not a reliable option. Meat and dairy were usually raised on an individual's farm. Meat, however, could be dried or smoked, allowing it to store for longer periods. Due to unsophisticated preservation, many other foods, including fruits and vegetables, were difficult to store through the winter unless pickled. Thus, during winter months, people ate larger portions of meat and dairy, and during the summer months, people ate larger portions of fruits and vegetables.

At this same time, there was great variety in the medical industry. Instead of physicians trained in one school of thought, each doctor could abide by his own philosophy and begin practicing with little to no formal training. While this allowed for an open market and a great deal of innovation and healing to take place, it also opened the door for conflicting information and methods that today seem questionable. Each doctor had a different philosophy and would use any number of herbs, medicines, foods, alcohol, and even poisons with patients. Lacking consistency and consensus, health care was a free-for-all. Some doctors, such as Samuel Thomson, developed life-altering herbal practices that Joseph Smith reportedly remarked were just as inspired as his introducing the restored gospel.[7]

---

[7] "Journal of Priddy Meeks," *Utah Historical Quarterly,* 1942, 10:145 p. 41.

Others, such as physician Benjamin Rush, a renowned and popular doctor of the day, began practicing extreme bleeding and purging to heal various ailments.[8]

Early Church Health and Nutrition Practices

As we previously mentioned, most Americans drank alcohol to varying degrees during this time, and the early Church leaders were no exception. But perhaps drinking wasn't the biggest problem among the brethren. Brigham Young explained what happened among the brethren when convening each day in the School of Prophets:

"[T]he first thing they did was to light their pipes, and, while smoking, talk about the great things of the kingdom, and spit all over the room, and as soon as the pipe was out of their mouths a large chew of tobacco would then be taken. Often when the Prophet entered the room to give the school instructions he would find himself in a cloud of tobacco smoke. This, and the complaints from his wife at having to clean so filthy a floor, made the Prophet think upon the matter, and he inquired of the Lord relating to the conduct of the elders in using tobacco, and the revelation known as the Word of Wisdom was the result."[9]

The whole situation was certainly less than ideal for those who were called of God as these elders were, especially when we remember that the room with the filthy floor was also Joseph's "translation room"—the same place where he often received revelations from God. For the Spirit of the Lord to instruct us, we must have cleanliness and order. Surely, Joseph must have had a difficult time obtaining the mind and will of the Lord under such circumstances. Joseph began inquiring of the Lord

---

[8] Robert L. North, "Benjamin Rush, MD: assassin or beloved healer?" *Baylor University Medical Center Proceedings*, January 2000.
[9] Brigham Young, *Journal of Discourses*, vol. 12, p. 158.

about what could be done, and on February 27, 1833, scarcely a month after the school started, he received the revelation later canonized as Doctrine and Covenants Section 89. This was the first revelation given in the School of Prophets, which is of great significance. The revelation was received while the brethren were congregated in the School of Prophets and was unanimously accepted by all in attendance. According to member Zebedee Coltrin, "When the Word of Wisdom was first presented by the Prophet Joseph. . . there were twenty out of the twenty-one who used tobacco and they all immediately threw their tobacco and pipes into the fire."[10]

The Word of Wisdom From 1834 to Today

Some Latter-day Saints in recent years have suggested that the Word of Wisdom was initially more of a set of guidelines rather than governing principles of health for Church members. This is because of the language in the text saying it was given "not by commandment."[11] However, the Prophet Joseph taught that members should not hold Church offices unless they lived the Word of Wisdom. He said: "No official member in this Church is worthy to hold an office after having the Word of Wisdom properly taught him; and he, the official member, neglecting to comply with and obey it."[12] As was the case so often with the Prophet, these were not just empty words. In 1838, David Whitmer was excommunicated from the Church on many charges, the first of which listed in Joseph's journal being for not observing the Word of Wisdom.[13]

We should note, however, that when the Word of Wisdom was given, it was understood to be principle-based, and thus, the application was not solely the letter of the law, but the spirit as

---

[10] Minutes, Salt Lake City School of Prophets, 3 Oct. 1883, p. 56.

[11] Doctrine and Covenants 89:2.

[12] Joseph Fielding Smith, *Teachings of the Prophet Joseph Smith*, (Salt Lake City, UT: Deseret Book 1976), p. 117.

[13] Joseph Smith, "The Scriptory Book–of Joseph Smith Jr.–President of the Church of Jesus Christ, of Latterday Saints In all the World," 13 April 1838, 31, The Joseph Smith Papers.

well. Namely, ensuring that agency and health of body and spirit were used as a framework for which one would determine a substance's use. This is why it was occasionally permitted for one to drink tea or use alcohol in certain circumstances. Overall it was clear that adherence to the Word of Wisdom was of utmost importance to the Saints and their membership in the Church.

In 1834, the Church Council officially declared an enduring policy that all Latter-Day Saints must obey the revelation to receive callings. It wasn't until the following year, in 1835, that the revelation known as the Word of Wisdom was published as Section 80 in the first edition of the Doctrine and Covenants.[14] In 1842, Hyrum Smith gave one of the most historic and first dedicated sermons on the Word of Wisdom in general conference, which we will draw from throughout this book.[15]

Although this revelation was not yet a binding commandment for the whole Church, members were still expected to adhere to the principles once taught, as Joseph explained. The Lord still expected obedience; nevertheless, He was patient with the Saints as they earnestly sought to remove bad habits from their lives, as He is with each of us.

After the death of the Prophet Joseph Smith and the subsequent migration of the Saints to Utah, Brigham Young often spoke passionately about and was an ardent supporter of the Word of Wisdom.[16] As evidence of his zeal for and devotion to the Word of Wisdom, President Young made a significant declaration and invitation to all Saints on September 9, 1851, some eighteen years after the revelation had been given. While the Patriarch to the Church, John Smith, delivered a talk in general conference on the Word of Wisdom, President Brigham Young arose and proposed that all Saints formally covenant to

---

[14] "Doctrine and Covenants, 1835," p. 207, The Joseph Smith Papers.
[15] "The Word of Wisdom," *Times and Seasons*, vol. 3, no. 15, 1 June 1842, p. 799.
[16] Brigham Young, *Journal of Discourses*, vol. 10, p. 202.

abstain from tea, coffee, tobacco, whiskey, and adhere to "all things mentioned in the Word of Wisdom."[17]

Many years later, President Spencer W. Kimball emphasized the fact that President Young gave the Word of Wisdom as a commandment when he said:

> "The Word of Wisdom is a commandment. In 1851 President Brigham Young gave to this Church the Word of Wisdom as a final and definite commandment. . . From 1851 until this day it is a commandment to all the members of the Church of Jesus Christ."[18]

It was during President Brigham Young's administration in the church that the Word of Wisdom was accepted as a binding commandment. As President Ezra Taft Benson taught:

> "At first the revelation was not given as a commandment. It was given as 'a principle with promise, adapted to the capacity of the weak and the weakest of all saints, who are or can be called saints.' This allowed time for the Saints to adjust to the principles contained in the revelation. In 1851, President Brigham Young proposed to the general conference of the Church that all Saints formally covenant to keep the Word of Wisdom. This proposal was unanimously upheld by the membership of the Church. Since that day, the revelation has been a binding commandment on all Church members."[19]

As we can see, the Word of Wisdom *did* become a binding commandment for the Church beginning with Brigham Young in 1851. However, just because it was then made a commandment doesn't mean that the consequences for non-compliance were

---

[17] "Minutes of the General Conference," *Millennial Star*, vol. 14, 1 February 1852, p. 35.
[18] Spencer W. Kimball, *The Teachings of Spencer W. Kimball*, (Salt Lake City, UT: Deseret Book Company, 1995), p. 201.
[19] Ezra Taft Benson, "A Principle With Promise," General Conference, April 1983.

immediately set forth. Even in 1898, President Wilford Woodruff declared that the Word of Wisdom must be strictly observed, but bishops ought not to withhold temple recommends from those who did not strictly adhere to it.[20]

In 1902, a mere 5 years later, President Joseph F. Smith urged stake presidents and bishops to refuse temple recommends to Saints who flagrantly violated the Word of Wisdom.[21] Ten years later he declared that middle-age men who have experience in the Church should not be ordained to the Priesthood nor recommended to the privileges of the House of the Lord unless they will abstain from the use of tobacco and intoxicating drinks.[22]

In the April 1931 General Conference, President Heber J. Grant in General Conference succinctly explained the issue of commandment vs. non-commandment:

> "I have met any number of people who have said the Word of Wisdom is not a command from the Lord, that it is not given by way of commandment. But the Word of Wisdom is the will of the Lord and the Lord says in the words that I have just read that it is not meet that we should be commanded in all things. . ."[23]

It wasn't until 1933 under President Grant, that the Word of Wisdom formally became a requirement to enter into the temple. However, as we have already discussed, the Word of Wisdom became a commandment in 1851 but was not a requirement for holding a temple recommend. It was in 1933 that the handbook of instructions for stake presidents and

---

[20] Historical Department journal history of the Church, 1830-2008; 1890-1899; 1898 May, Church History Library.

[21] Thomas G. Alexander, "The Word of Wisdom: From Principle to Requirement," *Dialogue: A Journal of Mormon Thought,* vol. 14, no. 3, 1981, 79.

[22] Anderson, Devery, *The Development of LDS Temple Worship, 1846-2000: A Documentary History,* (Salt Lake City, UT: Signature Books, 2011).

[23] Heber J. Grant, *Conference Report,* April 1931, pp. 12-13.

"hot drinks"—taught by Church leaders to refer specifically to tea and coffee."[28]

Interestingly enough, however, a careful reading of this statement will show that it does not contradict the statement made in 1972. It merely points out that caffeine is not specifically mentioned in Doctrine and Covenants 89.

The most recent clarifying statement from the Church came in August 2019 to include the use of many additional and increasingly common substances:

> "In recent publications for Church members, Church leaders have clarified that several substances are prohibited by the Word of Wisdom, including vaping or e-cigarettes, green tea, and coffee-based products. They also have cautioned that substances such as marijuana and opioids should be used only for medicinal purposes as prescribed by a competent physician."[29]

History in Perspective

What we have provided the reader in this chapter is certainly not a comprehensive history of the Word of Wisdom. Rather, it is a high-level perspective of how the revelation was lived and implemented since the time of the Prophet Joseph Smith. Perhaps the most important thing to remember with the Word of Wisdom is that it is a set of guiding principles. At the same time, we should also remember that even though the text says that it was not given as a commandment, it was given as the "will of God," which is effectively the same as a commandment. We need not worry over whether it was initially a commandment because, as we have already discussed, starting with Brigham Young it became a commandment—long before any one of us was alive. Of

---

[28] "Mormonism in the News: Getting It Right," The Newsroom Blog, Church of Jesus Christ of Latter-day Saints Newsroom, 29 August 2012.
[29] "Statement on the Word of Wisdom," Church of Jesus Christ of Latter-day Saints Newsroom, 15 August 2019.

course, there were varying levels of enforcement until it was made a requirement for temple attendance. Over the years, there have been clarifications and additions made by inspired prophets, but we would be wise to remember that we are not to be commanded in all things. The Brethren do not have to say something is specifically in violation of or in keeping with the Word of Wisdom for it to be so. Guided by the Spirit, we have the privilege and responsibility of seeking the spirit of the law. Perhaps President J. Reuben Clark, Jr. said it best:

> "The word of wisdom is not a rule of conduct; it is a law—the Lord's law—of health. It was promulgated by Him. The law existed before He told it to us; it would exist if the revelation were blotted out from the book. The Church authorities have nothing to do with the law. God, speaking through the forces of the physical world, has prescribed it, and so long as those forces exist the law will remain."[30]

In other words, the Word of Wisdom is not something we can decide for ourselves. It exists outside of the organization and authorities of the Church. By adhering to the principles, we place ourselves in a position to receive the natural consequences as well as the promises of the Lord.

---

[30] J. Reuben Clark, Jr., *Improvement Era*, vol. 36, November 1933, p. 806.

Chapter Three

Conspiring Men

*"And the Gentiles are lifted up in the pride of
their eyes, and . . . they put down the power
and miracles of God, and preach up unto
themselves their own wisdom and their own
learning, that they may get gain. . ."*

2 Nephi 26:20

The Purpose of the Word of Wisdom

Near the beginning of Doctrine and Covenants 89, the Lord
declares His purpose in revealing the Word of Wisdom:

> "In consequence of **evils and designs** which *do* and
> *will* exist in the hearts of **conspiring men** in the last
> days, I have warned you, and forewarn you, by giving
> unto you this word of wisdom by revelation."[1]

The Lord makes it clear that one of the main purposes of the
Word of Wisdom is to warn against the evil of conspiring men in
the last days. It is interesting to note that the Lord uses both the
terms warn and forewarn, implying that there were at the time
plans of evil concerning the health of man, but also that there
were plans yet to be concocted and implemented. For many of
us, this verse can feel somewhat nebulous as it is often hard to
understand or recognize what these secret combinations are,
how they operate, and why they would do such things. The

---

[1] Doctrine and Covenants 89:4, emphasis added.

purpose of this chapter is not to expose all of the past or present secret combinations that affect our health. Such an undertaking would require volumes. However, we do feel it is appropriate to dedicate a chapter to discussing the conspiring men and their influence over our health as the Lord has warned us in this revelation and throughout scripture.

Conspiring Men in the Scriptures and Early Church History

The beginning of conspiring men on the Earth can be traced back to when Cain made a covenant with Satan.[2] From Cain, these combinations and oaths were passed down from generation to generation to the point where they have existed "among all people."[3] What, exactly, is the purpose of these evil designs? The scriptures tell us plainly that they are built up to murder and "to get power and gain."[4] In more modern times, Brigham Young explained that the specific aim of many of these destructive groups has been to "lead astray every man and woman that wishes to be a latter-day saint."[5] The Book of Mormon is filled with examples of these types of associations seeking to lead astray and destroy for the purpose of amassing wealth and power. In Helaman, we learn that the Nephites began to support these evil works, beginning with the more wicked parts of society and then deceiving and convincing the more righteous part to "partake of their spoils."[6] The Book of Mormon makes clear that if upheld, secret combinations lead to pain and suffering of righteous individuals and the ultimate destruction of society.

In our own history, we know there were conspirators both in and out of the Church during the 1830s. Many attempts were made to poison an unsuspecting Joseph. In fact, on one

---

[2] Moses 5:29-32.
[3] Ether 8:20.
[4] Ether 11:15.
[5] Brigham Young, *Journal of Discourses*, vol. 8, page 344.
[6] Helaman 6:38.

occasion, they were nearly successful in killing the prophet and chipped one of his teeth in the process.[7] Another example of evils and designs by conspiring men was during the prophet's stay in Liberty Jail with other brethren. The verses in Doctrine and Covenants 121, revealed to the prophet during this difficult time, were deep and profound. While the Saints were being tormented and sorely persecuted in Missouri, the brethren in Liberty Jail also endured dire circumstances. It was recorded by several jailed with the prophet that they were subjected to eating human flesh.[8] As George A. Smith recounted, the guards withheld all but the "Mormon Beef" as they called it, and a little coffee or cornbread for nearly five days.[9] However, Joseph had received revelation for the brethren not to partake of the meat, sparing them from the sure sorrow that would have accompanied such a horrendous act.

Conspiring Men in Modern Times

One would hope that such evil would be done away with today, but it has only increased in severity and repugnance. One modern prophet boldly proclaimed that "[wickedness] is more highly organized, more cleverly disguised, and more powerfully promoted than ever before. Secret combinations lusting for power, gain, and glory are flourishing."[10]

There should be no question in the mind of the reader that nefarious works of the devil not only exist but run rampant in the world around us. We, as the latter-day Church, are not exempt from witnessing the secret combinations that exist today.

One of the most important things to remember to stay above the secret combinations threatening to destroy our health is that which sets us apart from Satan—our physical bodies. Satan never

---

[7] Joseph Smith, *History of the Church*, vol. 1, pp. 261-2.
[8] Hyrum Smith, *Times and Seasons*, vol. 4, p. 254.
[9] George A. Smith, *Journal of Discourses*, vol. 13, p. 108.
[10] Ezra Taft Benson, "I Testify," General Conference, October 1988.

had the opportunity to enter into this mortal probation and, as such, has never laid hold on a body of his own. He aims to get us to abuse our precious gift so that we might have enmity between us and our Creator. As we begin to understand this principle, it becomes clear why the Word of Wisdom so explicitly warns of conspiring men and outlines a clear path for us to keep our bodies safe in the face of these evil efforts. Satan, through his evil and destructive compacts, has inspired and recruited men to try and deceive us to get us to abuse and destroy our bodies so that we may be "miserable like unto [him]."[11]

On this very subject, Joseph Fielding Smith said, "One passage in [the Word of Wisdom] is quite generally overlooked. It states that the time should come when wicked and designing men would resort to **practices of adulteration of foods and drinks in order to get gain, to the injury and the health of their victims**. How true these words have been."[12] With this in mind, it is no wonder that the Lord revealed to the Prophet Joseph a code of health and a set of principles that would protect the Saints of the day and our own against the evils and designs that rage in the hearts of men, specifically concerning the constitution and maintenance of our bodies. It is not our intention to try and expose all of the corruption prevalent in the many food and health industries, but we do think it prudent to briefly discuss several particular industries that may fit under the term "conspiring men" that the Lord warned about.

Pharmakeia

As it has already been explained, since secret combinations and conspiring men have existed since Cain, it would be naive of us to think that conspiring men do not exist today. By nature, you will not often find these discussions in the spotlight or on the evening news–they wouldn't be called 'secret combinations'

---

[11] 2 Nephi 2:27.
[12] Joseph Fielding Smith, *Answers to Gospel Questions*, vol. 1, (Salt Lake City, UT: Deseret Book Company, 1957), p. 200.

if you could. However, the evidence is overwhelming. There may be no better example of conspiracy than in the health and wellness industry, a multi-trillion dollar enterprise.

The idea of conspiring men in the health industry is not a new concept. What may be shocking to many readers is that the Bible gives us hints about these conspirators. In the Greek version of the Bible, the word used whenever we see the word 'sorcery' in our English King James Version is 'pharmakeia,' which means "the use of medicine, drugs or spells."[13] It is interesting to note that the word pharmakeia is also the root for the words pharmaceuticals and pharmacy which are defined as "drugs" and "the preparation of drugs," respectively. In essence, mentions of sorceries in our King James Version of the Bible could be better understood when replaced with the term pharmakeia. For example, speaking of the last days, the Apostle John recorded in the book of Revelation:

> "And the rest of the men which were not killed by these plagues yet repented not of the works of their hands, that they should not worship devils, and idols of gold, and silver, and brass, and stone, and of wood: which neither can see, nor hear, nor walk: Neither repented they of their murders, nor of their sorceries (pharmakeia)."[14]

It is clear from these verses that those that have their hearts fixated upon the things of the world, including money, were also involved in murder and 'pharmakeia'. The reader will have to decide for himself or herself as to what this reference to pharmakeia could mean: medicine, drugs, or spells. However, John goes on to explain that the "merchants were the great men of the earth; for **by thy sorceries (pharmakeia) were all nations deceived**."[15]

---

[13] "G5331 - pharmakeia - Strong's Greek Lexicon (KJV)," *Blue Letter Bible*.
[14] Revelation 9:20-21.
[15] Revelation 18:23, emphasis added.

The additional insight provided by the Greek translation perhaps gives us a greater understanding as to the conspiracies that exist in the last days. Here, we have John the Revelator explaining that all of the nations of the earth would be deceived because of this 'pharmakeia.' Could it be that there are witches and wizards throughout the world using sorcery to cast magic and spells, deceiving the world? Maybe. But would it not be far more logical to believe that John is referencing an industry that is hiding in plain sight such as the pharmaceutical industry? The hope and promise of modern medicine are to become well and be made whole, but is this promise being fulfilled?

Consider the following: Disease rates have skyrocketed over the last 50 years. Studies show that chronic disease in the United States has *more than doubled* in the last 20 years alone.[16] According to the most recent data, over 60 percent of the population have at least one chronic disease.[17] Chronic diseases are also responsible for an estimated seven out of every 10 deaths in the United States, killing over 2 million Americans each year alone.[18] By contrast, in the year 1900, disease or illness of any kind accounted for five out of every 10 deaths killing only 204,992 people altogether.[19] What's more is that according to an estimate from Johns Hopkins University, medical errors in hospitals are the third leading cause of death in the United States, killing an estimated 400,000 annually.[20] To put this into

---

[16] Sarah Wild et al., "Global prevalence of diabetes: estimates for the year 2000 and projections for 2030," *Diabetes care*, vol. 27, no. 5, 2004, pp. 1047-53.

[17] "Chronic Diseases in America," Centers for Disease Control and Prevention, https://www.cdc.gov/chronicdisease/resources/infographic/chronic-diseases.htm.

[18] Melonie Heron, "Deaths: Leading Causes for 2017," National Vital Statistics Report, vol. 68, no. 6, p. 12.

[19] "Leading Causes of Death, 1900-1998," Centers for Disease Control and Prevention, p. 67, https://www.cdc.gov/nchs/data/dvs/lead1900_98.pdf.

[20] Martin A Makary and Michael Daniel, "Medical error—the third leading cause of death in the US," *BMJ 2016*; 353 :i2139.

perspective, more people die annually these days at the hands of medical error than all of the combined deaths in the year 1900.[21]

This data indicates that disease rates and deaths have risen significantly, despite drastic increases in healthcare spending and a perceived overall improvement in healthcare quality. Researchers have suggested that life expectancy is on the *decline* and the Millennial generation may be the first to live shorter and less healthy lives than their parents.[22] All of this, yet in the United States per capita health care spending exceeds $10,000 a year, and disease rates continue to skyrocket.[23]

Perhaps the greatest evidence for 'pharmakeia' or conspiring men in the pharmaceutical industry is the opioid crisis in America, and the awful role it has played in our national health. For example, from 1991 to 2013 the number of prescriptions for opioids more than doubled from 76 million to 207 million.[24] Correspondingly, there has been a significant increase in opioid addiction and deaths.

The most current data from 2012 indicates that at that time, 2.1 million people per day were abusing opioids in the United States alone. From 1999 to 2012 the number of unintended opioid overdose deaths quadrupled.[25] These deaths account for more than 67 percent of total drug overdose deaths.[26] Surely the figures today would be much more sobering. It seems that

[21] "Leading Causes of Death, 1900-1998," Centers for Disease Control and Prevention, p. 67, https://www.cdc.gov/nchs/data/dvs/lead1900_98.pdf.

[22] S. Jay Olshansky et al., "A Potential Decline in Life Expectancy in the United States in the 21st Century," *The New England Journal of Medicine*, vol. 352, no. 11, 2005, pp. 1138-45.

[23] Bradley Sawyer and Cynthia Cox, "How does health spending in the U.S. compare to other countries?," Peterson Center on Healthcare and Kaiser Family Foundation, Health System Tracker, 7 December 2018.

[24] International Narcotics Control Board Report 2008, United Nations Pubns. 2009. p. 20.

[25] Pradip et al, "Associations of Nonmedical Pain Reliever Use and Initiation of Heroin Use in the US," Center for behavioral Health Statistics and QualityData Review, SAMHSA, 2013.

[26] FB Ahmad et al., "Provisional drug overdose death counts," National Center for Health Statistics. 2020.

everywhere you look, lawsuits are piling up regarding medical malpractice and opioids.[27] In fact, as we were writing this book in 2020, a prominent doctor pleaded guilty to opioid conspiracy and healthcare fraud.[28]

As if this wasn't enough, pharmaceutical companies are some of the largest donors to members of Congress, irrespective of political party.[29] If this 'pharmakeia' that John speaks of is the pharmaceutical industry, commonly referred to as 'Big Pharma' (which should be an indication in and of itself), we ought to consider the implications. None of this is to suggest that everyone involved in pharmaceuticals or the medical industry is evil or conspiring, but these are important points that we should keep in mind when it comes to our health. What we ought to give more attention to, however, is what the Lord has said concerning healing. We will discuss this in greater detail in a later chapter.

Smoking

If you lived between the 1920s and 1950s, smoking was glamorous. Actors, athletes, politicians, and doctors alike were avid proponents of smoking.[30] It appeared on the screen, on billboards, in magazines, and over the airwaves. During this time the average per capita consumption was 4,000 cigarettes per year or an average of 10.9 cigarettes per day.[31] If you weren't smoking, you clearly didn't understand the health trends of the day. Though it may be hard for us to comprehend now, doctors

---

[27] "Several charged in $9.6 million opioid distribution conspiracy," United States Drug Enforcement Agency, 1 June 2018, Press Release.

[28] "Doctor Pleads Guilty to Opioid Conspiracy and Health Care Fraud," United States Department of Justice, U.S. Attorney's Office, Eastern District of Virginia, 4 May 2020, Press Release.

[29] Adriana Belmonte, "FDA medical adviser: 'Congress is owned by pharma'," Yahoo Finance, 13 March 2019.

[30] Stuart Elliot, "When Doctors, and Even Santa, Endorsed Tobacco," The New York Times, 6 October 2008.

[31] Centers for Disease Control and Prevention. CDC Surveillance Summaries, November 18, 1994. MMWR 1994;43(No. SS-3).

exclusively for the rich and powerful. It wasn't until the 1800s that the slave trade brought refined sugar into the world market.

Beginning in the 1950s and 1960s, many began to question sugar and its impact on health.[43] Many began to believe that perhaps sugar was to blame for the rise of health issues plaguing the nation. Studies began to be conducted to determine the reality of this potential link. In 1965, one of the biggest studies on sugar was conducted.[44] Unfortunately for the general public, the funding for these studies came from the sugar industry itself. This study found that sucrose was directly linked to an increased risk of heart disease. Rather than admit the finding, which would have been quite a blow, the industry did what was necessary to survive: they buried it. The study never saw the light of day, and the general public didn't find out until decades later. Not only did the sugar industry hide the study, but over the past few years it was discovered that they *paid* researchers to link heart disease to fat and downplay the role of sugar.[45]

While this instance is shocking, it is certainly not uncommon. For instance, one of the top funders in the world for health studies is Coca Cola.[46] If they are consistently funding the studies, what do you think the outcomes will be? Perhaps this is why we still see studies promoting the alleged health benefits of soda consumption.[47] However, a massive body of evidence

---

[43] Camila Domonoske, "50 Years Ago, Sugar Industry Quietly Paid Scientists To Point Blame At Fat," NPR, 13 September 2016.

[44] Kearns CE, Schmidt LA, Glantz SA, "Sugar Industry and Coronary Heart Disease Research: A Historical Analysis of Internal Industry Documents," *JAMA Internal Medicine,* vol. 176, no. 11 2016, pp. 1680–1685.

[45] Ibid.

[46] Nicole Westman, "Coca-Cola funds health research-and can kill the studies it doesn't like," Popular Science, 10 May 2019.

[47] J.C Peters et al., "The effects of water and non-nutritive sweetened beverages on weight loss during a 12-week weight loss treatment program," *Obesity,* vol. 22, 2014, pp. 1415-21.

suggests the contrary, specifically regarding the kind of sugar promoted by Coca-Cola.[48]

To further complicate things, today there are over 69 different legal names for this refined sugar product–names which one may not recognize or associate with sugar.[49] Some of these names include High Fructose Corn Syrup, Glucose solids, Maltodextrin, Maltose, Mannitol, Ethyl maltol, Fructose, Galactose, Treacle, and many more. Is it any wonder that we are confused at the grocery store and can hardly find a product that isn't laced with, or even bathed in, sugar? From ketchup to soups, there is sugar hidden in nearly every processed food on the market. This is one of many reasons it is estimated that 30-40 percent of all healthcare expenditures in the US go to health issues directly linked with excess consumption of sugar.[50]

Even with all of this data a question remains–is sugar *that* bad for our spirits? The answer to this question comes to us from the creation story when the Lord commands Adam and Eve to eat fruit as their primary food source.[51] Fruit is the food that God has ordained for us; it is naturally sweet and satiating. It is also interesting to note that mothers' milk has a sweet taste. Breast milk, for most of human history, was the only food that a child would taste for the first years of life. Is it any wonder that after only drinking this sweet life-giving nectar for months, that the child would then develop a permanent desire for sweet foods?

The Lord gave each of us an inherent desire for sweet things, which is apparent in our ability to see color and taste sweet things that most animals do not have.[52] Moreover, carbohydrates

---

[48] Joe Leech, "13 Ways That Sugary Soda Is Bad for Your Health," Healthline, 8 February 2019.

[49] Jennifer L. Pomeranz, "The Bittersweet Truth About Sugar Labeling Regulations: They Are Achievable and Overdue," *American Journal of Public Health*, vol. 102, no. 7, 2012, pp. e14-20.

[50] "Sugar Consumption at a crossroads," Credit Suisse Research Institute, September 2013, p. 38.

[51] Moses 2:29.

[52] Heather Hatfield, "The Science Behind How We Taste," WebMD, 16 May 2005.

are essential to our health in many ways.[53] However, we know that Satan is a skillful imitator. As President Ezra Taft Benson said:

> "Whenever the God of Heaven establishes by revelation his design, Satan always comes among men to pervert the doctrine, saying, 'Believe it not.' He often establishes a counterfeit system, designed to deceive the children of men."[54]

Is it any wonder that Satan would want to pervert our natural, God-given sweet tooth with a nefarious counterfeit, namely refined sugar? By removing the good and healthful parts of the fruit you are left with the extracted, concentrated, and deliciously sweet sugar content. Sugar triggers the opiate receptors of the brain which stimulate the pleasure centers even *more* than cocaine, making it highly addictive.[55] Because of this, many become reliant upon it to be happy and satiated. Researchers indicate that it is often easier to break drug addictions than sugar addictions.[56] Unlike man's laboratory invention, God's natural creation does not subject and trick our natural desires for that which is sweet, but rather it fulfills.

Wheat

We will talk more about wheat and, more broadly, grains in the chapter about the 'Dos' of the Word of Wisdom, but this aspect of Doctrine and Covenants 89 has always been interesting to the writers, specifically Cassidy. In part, because I (Cassidy) was diagnosed with a rare but severe gluten allergy years ago,

---

[53] "Carbohydrates," The Nutrition Source, Harvard School of Public Health, 22 May 2019.

[54] Ezra Taft Benson, "A Vision and a Hope for the Youth of Zion," BYU Devotional, 12 April 1977.

[55] David J. Mysels and Maria A Sullivan. "The relationship between opioid and sugar intake: review of evidence and clinical applications." Journal of opioid management vol. 6, no. 6, 2010, pp. 445-52.

[56] Serge H Ahmed et al. "Sugar addiction: pushing the drug-sugar analogy to the limit." *Current opinion in clinical nutrition and metabolic care*, vol. 16, no. 4, 2013, pp. 434-9.

similar to Celiac. Since then, I have had to stay far away from products like wheat, rye, barley, and regular oats. As I began studying the Word of Wisdom, I became frustrated with the fact that I was allergic to a food the Lord commands to be the "staff of life." I have met countless others throughout the years that verbalize the same concerns. This led me to conduct a serious investigation into the origins of wheat and the changes it has undergone throughout time. What I found was shocking.

Wheat has been a staple of nearly every civilization's diet as evidenced throughout the Bible, Book of Mormon, and other historical records. And yet, wheat allergies have increased by over 500 percent in the last 50 years.[57] How is it possible for such a staple food to turn into such a high allergenic food? As Dr. William Davis indicated, today's "wheat isn't even wheat, thanks to some of the most intense cross breeding efforts ever seen. The wheat products sold to you today are nothing like the wheat products of our grandmother's age, very different from the wheat of the early 20th century, and completely transformed from the wheat of the Bible and earlier."[58]

Throughout time, various combinations of seeds were combined in a process called hybridization.[59] These seeds were hybridized for more effective crop yields and to create new varieties. However, starting in the 1960s this hybridization took a dramatic turn. In new genetic experiments, researchers discovered that they could make wheat that would contain pesticides naturally in the seed itself which would increase crop yield.[60] Since this time, wheat has undergone such a change that it is hardly recognizable. It is modified to contain chemicals that

---

[57] Carlo Catassi et al., "Diagnosis of Non-Celiac Gluten Sensitivity (NCGS): The Salerno Experts' Criteria." Nutrients vol. 7, no. 6, 18 June 2015, pp. 4966-77.
[58] "Modern Wheat Really Isn't Wheat At All," PreventDisease.com, 16 January, 2012.
[59] M. Florian Mette et al., "Hybrid Breeding in Wheat," *Advances in Wheat Genetics: From Genome to Field,* 2015, pp. 225-32.
[60] Ibid.

improve yield but are toxic to humans.[61] Furthermore, bioengineers use Glyphosate, a key ingredient used in RoundUp Weed Killer to spray the crops while growing.[62] They also use it as a drying agent. Glyphosate is highly carcinogenic and has been linked to multiple modern health issues.[63] And yet, our wheat contains it in the seeds, is sprayed with it in the field, and is dried with it.

But it gets even worse: a vast majority of wheat products on the market are highly processed. Leaving out the bran and germ, which contain 80 percent of the nutrients, these make for fluffy and addicting baked goods but wreak havoc on digestion, hormones, and other bodily processes.[64] Even products that are labeled "100% wheat" are misleading because the wheat is already contaminated with chemicals and irradiated with gamma rays and high-dose X-rays to induce mutations.[65]

It may sound depressing that the food which should be our "staff of life" has been so abused and changed. But should it be any surprise that the food the Lord commands we should eat most has become one of the adulterated foods that Joseph Fielding Smith said conspiring men would create? Lucky for us, hope is not lost. Wheat is classified under the genus (or plant family) Triticum. Under this umbrella, there are over 30,000 varieties of wheat.[66] When we think of wheat, we often think of

---

[61] Robin Mesnage et al., "Major pesticides are more toxic to human cells than their declared active principles," *BioMed research international*, vol. 2014, 2014.

[62] C.M. Benbrook, "Trends in glyphosate herbicide use in the United States and globally," *Environ Sci Eur,* vol. 28, no. 3, 2016.

[63] Siriporn Thongprakaisang et al., "Glyphosate induces human breast cancer cells growth via estrogen receptors," *Food and Chemical Toxicology*, vol. 59, 2013, pp. 129-36.

[64] Dawei Yan et al., "The Functions of the Endosperm During Seed Germination," *Plant and Cell Physiology*, vol. 55, no. 9, September 2014, pp. 1521–33.

[65] Melki Mongi and A. Marouani, "Effects of gamma rays irradiation on seed germination and growth of hard wheat," *Environmental Chemistry Letters,* vol. 8, pp. 307-10.

[66] Elieser S. Posner, "Wheat flour milling" American Association of Cereal Chemists, 2011.

the 1 or 2 varieties that have been altered. Do we think of all of the other grains that have existed for thousands of years and have remained unadulterated by the hand of man? It simply doesn't make sense to consume this wheat-like product that has been hybridized time and time again, modified to contain glyphosate in its seeds, sprayed with more carcinogens after being picked, removed of its bran and germ, and then mixed with toxic trace substances so it can meet the FDA standards.[67] Most importantly, however, is the fact that the Lord does not approve of this kind of hybridizing. In the Old Testament, He plainly says "thou shalt not sow thy field with **mingled seed**.[68] . ." The Prophet Joseph Smith even hinted at this when he wrote in his journal:

> "God has made certain decrees which are fixed, and immovable, for instance; God set the sun, the moon, and the stars in the heavens; and gave them their laws, conditions and bounds which they cannot pass, **except by his commandments** . . . God has set many signs on the Earth, as well as in the heavens . . . the fruit of the tree, the herb of the field; all bear a sign that seed hath been planted there; for it is a decree of the Lord that every tree, plant, and herb bearing seed, **should bring forth of its kind, and cannot come forth after any other law, or principle**."[69]

With the evidence stacking up and the Lord weighing in on the matter, it should be clear that these man-made, hybridized foods are not of God and not good for our bodies.

---

[67] P. K. Newby et al., "Intake Of Whole Grains, Refined Grains, And Cereal Fiber Measured With 7-D Diet Records And Associations With Risk Factors For Chronic Disease," *American Journal of Clinical Nutrition*, vol. 86, no. 2007, March 2017, pp. 1745-53.

[68] Leviticus 19:19, emphasis added.

[69] "History, 1838–1856, volume C-1 [2 November 1838–31 July 1842]," p. 1296, The Joseph Smith Papers, emphasis added.

God's Answer to Conspiring Men in the Last Days

The Lord knew that all of these things would come to pass in the days preceding His Second Coming. Indeed, He knew of the "evils and designs" that rage in the hearts of men for power and personal profit. Today, there is so much information and confusion when it comes to our health, and unfortunately, there are consequences for following bad information. It is for this very reason that the Lord provided the Word of Wisdom, and we ought to pursue a careful examination of it.

It should be noted that what conspiring men do is complex and difficult for the masses to understand. This helps the few "experts" wield authority and power over the many of society, often going unchallenged or unquestioned. What God does is simple and plain for all to understand, each according to his own level of understanding. The information is readily available to all who will seek. The Word of Wisdom is no different. The world would have us believe that things just happen to our health and there is often no answer or solution. We disagree with that assertion. We have experienced the health and healing that comes by living the principles found in the Word of Wisdom and by forgoing the philosophies of men, even when we were told that hope and healing were impossible.

Chapter Four

The 'Don'ts'

*"The elements are the tabernacle of God; yea,
man is the tabernacle of God, even temples;
and whatsoever temple is defiled, God shall
destroy that temple."*
Doctrine and Covenants 93:35

The List of Don'ts

For many members of the Church, a discussion of the Word
of Wisdom often entails a narrow, simple list of "don'ts"
contained within the revelation and the later statements made
by modern prophets. For some of us, this is where the revelation
begins and ends. These items include hot drinks, strong drinks,
wine, tobacco, as well as drugs. As we previously discussed in
chapter two, most of these items were frequently consumed
during the time in which the revelation was given. This was a
major adjustment for most members, and still stands as a major
dividing line between members of the Church and the rest of the
world.

One of the incredible aspects of our time is that new evidence
has shown each of these items is not only an excitotoxin and
stimulant, but they are addictive and lead to poor health
outcomes as well.[1] Despite this evidence, however, much of the
mainstream medical and dietary advice still advocates for

---

[1] Manev, H et al. "Delayed increase of Ca2+ influx elicited by glutamate: role in
neuronal death." *Molecular pharmacology* vol. 36,1 (1989), p. 106-12.

'moderate' or 'healthy' consumption of each of these items.[2] Yet, many Saints have seen innumerable blessings from abstaining.

Hot Drinks

There are some in the Church who have justified their use of various beverages based on the general nature of the term "hot drinks." However, the Church has offered a clear stance on this since the revelation was given. In the first-ever General Conference talk dedicated to the Word of Wisdom, Joseph Smith clearly explained that the term hot drinks was specifically referring to tea and coffee.[3] Hyrum Smith echoed those words in his 1842 Conference sermon dedicated to the Word of Wisdom. The Church has reiterated this position over and over again, most recently included in the August 2019 official statement on the Word of Wisdom.[4]

Many may assume that because tea has historically been singled out, that all tea–including herbal tea–should be avoided. However, there are important nuances to consider. The tea referred to in the Word of Wisdom (as specified by modern prophets) is derived from the leaves of a single plant–the tea bush, also called *camellia sinensis*. Green tea, black tea, white tea, and oolong tea are the teas that come from this plant. The only difference is how they are processed. Herbal teas, as the name implies, are produced from any number of different herbs. Herbal teas are not even tea at all. Technically, they are either an infusion or decoction, depending on how they are prepared. Unlike real tea (which can only be brewed from leaves of the tea bush), herbal teas are prepared from steeping the leaves, stems, flowers, roots, bark, or rhizomes of herbs. Therefore, the admonition to avoid tea refers only to green tea, black tea, white

---

[2] Kris Gunnars, "Why Is Coffee Good for You? Here Are 7 Reasons," Healthline, 30 April 2018.

[3] Joel H. Johnson, *Voice from the Mountains*, (Salt Lake City: Juvenile Instructor Office, 1881), p. 12.

[4] "Statement on the Word of Wisdom," Church of Jesus Christ of Latter-day Saints Newsroom, 15 August 2019.

tea, and oolong tea.[5] Herbal infusions (better known as herbal tea) are different products altogether.

Though it is clear that coffee and tea are two of the primary substances that are to be avoided, many are shocked to learn that the word "hot" could cover many other beverages as well. The word "hot" could refer to the actual temperature of the drink, as hot drinks have negative impacts on the esophagus and on digestion,[6] in which case any kind of hot drink such as cider, chocolate, or even herbal tea would be out of the question if consumed while hot. However, one of the most important things to keep in mind when it comes to studying the scriptures is to take into account what the words meant when they were written. Language changes over time and words often lose meaning. By looking at scriptural definitions rather than modern definitions, we can better understand what the Lord means. In 1828, Noah Webster published the *American Dictionary of the English Language*, considered by many to be the most authoritative dictionary concerning the King James Bible and early 19th century America. In this dictionary, "hot" could be defined as relating to temperature, but it could also be defined as: "stimulating; or pungent."[7] The word stimulating serves as a springboard from which we can begin to understand what the Lord intended with this specific directive. Related to this very definition, George Q. Cannon remarked that chocolate, cocoa, and all drinks of that kind are considered "hot drinks" and should be avoided.[8]

This definition seems to indicate that there are a variety of other beverages that are enervating that fit within the realm of "hot drinks" while not often discussed. Caffeinated soda drinks are one such example. While the Church has never taken an

---

[5] Victor L. Ludlow, *Principles and Practices of the Restored Gospel*, (Salt Lake City, UT: Deseret Book Company 2011), p. 434.

[6] Dana Loomis et al., "Carcinogenicity of drinking coffee, mate, and very hot beverages," *The Lancet*, vol. 17, no. 7, pp. 877-8.

[7] Noah Webster, "hot," *An American Dictionary of the English Language*, 1828.

[8] George Q. Cannon, *Journal of Discourses*, vol. 12, p. 221.

official position on soda, there have been several statements made by prophets that give us insight worthy of our consideration.

For example, in the 1922 General Conference, President Heber J. Grant said, referring to the Saints having sung "We Thank Thee O God For a Prophet" at the conference:

> "Now, if you mean it—I am not going to give any command, but I will ask it as a personal, individual favor to me, to let coca-cola alone. There are plenty of other things you can get at the soda fountains without drinking that which is injurious. The Lord does not want you to use any drug that creates an appetite for itself."[9]

Another similar admonition came from President Spencer W. Kimball who taught: "I never drink any of the cola drinks and my personal hope would be that no one would."[10] Yet another prophet, namely Howard W. Hunter, added similar counsel in conjunction with striving to live the spirit of the law rather than only the letter:

> "**Live the spirit of the Word of Wisdom**. We complicate the simplicity of the Word of Wisdom. The Lord said don't drink tea, coffee, or use tobacco or liquor and that admonition is simple. But we confuse it by asking if cola drinks are against the Word of Wisdom. The 89th Section of the Doctrine and Covenants doesn't say anything about cola drinks, but we ask questions that go beyond the simplicity of the lesson that has been taught. We know that caffeine is taken out of coffee and used as an ingredient of cola drinks. It seems to me that if we probably want to live the spirit of the law we

---

[9] Heber J. Grant, *Conference Report*, April 1922, p. 165.
[10] Spencer W. Kimball, *Teachings of Spencer W. Kimball*, edited by Edward L. Kimball, (Salt Lake City: Bookcraft, 1982), p. 202.

probably wouldn't partake of that which had been taken from what we were told not to drink."[11]

If soda drinks are injurious and the brethren have previously advised against its use, it would seem that the same principle would include even more damaging and toxic products of recent invention such as energy drinks and other drinks intended to stimulate the brain. If we consider the definition of "hot" from 1828, a frozen can of "Monster Energy Drink" would be much more of a "hot" drink than a freshly-made, hot cup of coffee, as it is far more stimulating.

Speaking on the use of stimulating drinks, Brigham Young taught the Saints what they *should* drink saying, "It is difficult to find anything more healthy to drink than good cold water, such as flows down to us from springs and snows of our mountains. **This is the beverage we should drink**. It should be our drink at all times."[12]

Though many already know the risks associated with the consumption of many of our modern stimulating drinks, a reminder certainly serves us well. There is no reliable study or good data that suggests caffeine is good for long term health, though headlines would have you believe otherwise.[13] Soda consumption, for instance, is associated with Leukemia, non-Hodgkin's lymphoma, and multiple myeloma.[14] It is also linked with diabetes, heart disease, and cancer–the top killers in the world.[15] Perhaps the most telling data indicates that soda

---

[11] Howard W. Hunter, *Teachings of Howard W. Hunter*, (Salt Lake City, UT: Deseret Book Company, 1997), pp. 104-5, emphasis added.
[12] John A. Widtsoe, *Discourses of Brigham Young*, (Salt Lake City, UT: Deseret Book Company, 1951), p. 187, emphasis added.
[13] Ted Kallmyer, "20+ Harmful Effects of Caffeine," Caffeine Informer, 29 May 2020.
[14] Eva S. Schernhammer et al., "Consumption of artificial sweetener- and sugar-containing soda and risk of lymphoma and leukemia in men and women." *The American journal of clinical nutrition*, vol. 96, no. 6 (2012), pp. 1419-28.
[15] Noel T. Mueller et al., "Soft Drink and Juice Consumption and Risk of Pancreatic Cancer: The Singapore Chinese Health Study," *Cancer*

drinkers have decreased longevity and accelerated cell aging.[16] However, soda isn't the only beverage linked with health risks. Coffee and tea have also been found to increase hypertension and increase the risk of a heart attack four fold.[17] Studies have found that tea and coffee lead to increased instances of breast disease.[18] Additionally, caffeine has been shown to lead to increased anxiety, depression, and medication usage.[19] These stimulating, caffeinated drinks would surely be categorized as "hot" according to Webster were they around in the 1830s. Furthermore, modern research has shown that they can do great harm to the body. Our use of such substances would be worthy of examination.

Strong Drinks and Wine

Perhaps the most widely understood aspect of the Word of Wisdom is the avoidance of alcohol. The idea of abstaining from alcohol is biblical in nature. The book of Proverbs reminds us: "It is not for kings to drink wine; nor for princes strong drink."[20] Also in the Bible, we are reminded that it is a sin to be drunk and to give your neighbor drink.[21] Even Isaiah gives a warning to those that drink.[22]

Epidemiology, Biomarkers & Prevention, vol. 19, no. 2 (2010), pp. 447-55. See also Vasanti S. Malik et al., "Sugar-Sweetened Beverages, Obesity, Type 2 Diabetes Mellitus, and Cardiovascular Disease Risk," Circulation, vol. 121, no. 11 (2010), pp. 1356-64.

[16] Cindy W. Leung et al., "Soda and cell aging: associations between sugar-sweetened beverage consumption and leukocyte telomere length in healthy adults from the National Health and Nutrition Examination Surveys," American journal of public health, vol. 104, no. 12 (2014): pp. 2425-31.

[17] "Coffee linked with increased cardiovascular risk in young adults with mild hypertension," European Society of Cardiology, 29 August 2015, Press Release.

[18] Coleen A. Boyle et al., "Caffeine Consumption and Fibrocystic Breast Disease: A Case-Control Epidemiologic Study," Journal of the National Cancer Institute, vol. 72, no. 5 1984, pp. 1015-19.

[19] D. M. Veleber and D. I. Templer, "Effects of caffeine on anxiety and depression," Journal of Abnormal Psychology, vol. 93, no. 1 1984, pp. 120-22.

[20] Proverbs 31:4–5.

[21] Habakkuk 2:15.

[22] Isaiah 5:22.

Until the early 1900s wine was used in the Lord's Church for a sacrament. Christ is said to have drank wine when he lived on this earth, and He commanded Joseph Smith to use wine for the sacrament. It is important to note, as John A. Widstoe suggests, "the 'pure wine' in Doctrine and Covenants 89:6 is understood to mean new or unfermented grape juice."[23] However, since 1906 under President Joseph F. Smith, the Church has abolished the use of wine in any capacity.[24]

The word "wine" in the Bible is a generic term; sometimes it means grape juice and other times it meant alcoholic beverages.[25] Historians have indicated that the Jews and other nations in the Biblical world used wine that was often unfermented and normally mixed with water.[26] One text indicated that the wine in Biblical times was "unfermented or fermented stored wine diluted with water at a ratio as high as 20 to 1."[27] However, even a much lower ratio of three to one water-diluted, wine would affect the bladder long before it became intoxicating to the mind.[28]

Regardless of the arguments in favor of the use of alcohol in the Lord's Church, there are precedents for abstinence. There are multiple examples in the scriptures of the Lord's covenant people being commanded to forgo alcohol. The Nazarites are one such group. The Nazarites were people who dedicated themselves to the Lord and received protection as long as they did not partake of any wine or fermented drink and did not cut

---

[23] John A. Widtsoe and Leah D. Widtsoe, *The Word of Wisdom A Modern Interpretation*, (Salt Lake City, UT: Deseret Book Company 1950), pp. 60–61.

[24] Thomas G. Alexander, "The Word of Wisdom: From Principle to Requirement," *Dialogue: A Journal of Mormon Thought* vol. 14, no. 3 1981, p. 79.

[25] See Deuteronomy 11:14; 2 Chronicles 31:5; Nephi 13:15; Proverbs 3:10; Isaiah 16:10; 65:8; 1 Timothy 5:23.

[26] A. R. S. Kennedy, "Wine and Strong Drink," Dictionary of the Bible, rev. ed. (New York, NY: Scribner's, 1963) pp. 1038-39.

[27] Bob Stein, "Wine Drinking in New Testament Times," *Christianity Today,* vol. 19, 20 June 1975, pp. 10-11.

[28] Ibid.

their hair.[29] In the book of Leviticus, we also learn that Aaron and other priests were commanded, "Do not drink wine nor strong drink, thou, nor thy sons with thee" that they would be examples of the "difference between holy and unholy, and between unclean and clean".[30] The command in modern days is not unprecedented, as it was also commanded in biblical times.

Alcohol, perhaps more than nearly any other substance examined in the Word of Wisdom, limits one's agency. While intoxicated, proper use of agency is impaired and people may do things contrary to their natural and spiritual inclinations. As President Russell M. Nelson has reminded us, agency is the thing that Satan envies the most; he will do anything in his power to get us to abuse ours.[31] Similarly, President J. Reuben Clark said:

> "Over the earth ... the demon drink is in control. Drunken with strong drink, men have lost their reason; their counsel has been destroyed; their judgment and vision are fled; they reel forward to destruction. Drink brings cruelty into the home; it walks arm in arm with poverty; its companions are disease and plague; it puts chastity to flight; and it knows neither honesty nor fair dealing; it is a total stranger to truth; it drowns conscience; it is the bodyguard of evil; it curses all who touch it. Drink has brought more woe and misery, broken more hearts, wrecked more homes, committed more crimes, filled more coffins than all the wars the world has suffered."[32]

Even in small amounts, alcohol changes the function of our brains. Studies show that just one alcoholic drink can cause blurred vision, slurred speech, slower reaction times, impaired

---

[29] Numbers 6:3, 4.
[30] Leviticus 10: 8-10.
[31] Russell M. Nelson, "Addiction or Freedom," General Conference, October 1988.
[32] J. Reuben Clark Jr., *Conference Report*, October 1942, p. 8.

memory, and a loss of balance.[33] Additionally, alcohol consumption, even at very low levels, is linked with breast and prostate cancer.[34] It is also linked with high blood pressure, liver cirrhosis (damage to liver cells), and pancreatitis (inflammation of the pancreas).[35]

Though it is clear that alcohol is not to be consumed internally, it still has a place in our health regimen. According to Doctrine and Covenants 89 verse 7, its intended use is "for the washing of your bodies." Alcohol is an effective and useful treatment for cleansing wounds and abrasions. When alcohol is used on the skin for treatment, it is fulfilling its intended purpose.[36]

Tobacco

For many of us, tobacco is not a temptation. It has a potent smell, is messy, and has a strong taste. However, it is extremely addictive.[37] Anyone who has overcome this addiction can tell you just how difficult it can be. Perhaps that is the danger of tobacco products. They are made to bring the user back for more and more. The addictive nature of tobacco is what should be of greatest concern to us because it "interfere[s] with the delicate feelings of spiritual communication."[38] President George Albert Smith points out that although tobacco may not seem like a big deal to some people, it has "been the means of destroying their spiritual life, has been the means of driving from them the companionship of the Spirit of our Father, has alienated them

---

[33] "Alcohol's Damaging Effects on the Brain," *Alcohol Alert*, U.S. Department of Health and Human Services, no. 63, 2004.

[34] "Alcohol Use and Cancer," American Cancer Society, 9 June 2020.

[35] H Joe Wang et al., "Alcohol, inflammation, and gut-liver-brain interactions in tissue damage and disease development." *World journal of gastroenterology*, vol. 16, no. 11 2010, pp. 1304-13.

[36] "Section 89, The Word of Wisdom," Doctrine and Covenants Student Manual, 2002, pp. 206–11.

[37] "The Health Consequences of Smoking—50 Years of Progress: A Report of the Surgeon General," Centers for Disease Control and Prevention, 2014.

[38] Boyd K. Packer, "Personal Revelation: The Gift, the Test, and the Promise," General Conference, October 1994.

from the society of good men and women, and has brought upon them the disregard and reproach of the children that have been born to them."[39] There should be no doubt that tobacco is both addictive and harmful.

As we discussed in the previous chapter, tobacco has historically been glamorized and promoted by many as a healthy choice. Evidence now indicates that tobacco is not only detrimental to health but can also be deadly. The mortality rate for tobacco users is three times higher than nonusers.[40] Tobacco, in any form, is linked to a significant increase in heart attack.[41] The most popular form of tobacco, smoking, is perhaps the most frightening form. Cigarettes contain over 600 ingredients, many of which are incredibly harmful to the body.[42] When combined in cigarettes, they produce over 4,000 chemical compounds, 69 of which are carcinogenic.[43] To say that cigarettes and other forms of tobacco are harmful is an understatement.

However, similar to alcohol, tobacco has great medicinal value when used externally on wounds and bruises.[44] Many great herbalists use tobacco leaves externally for a number of ailments. As the text of Section 89 indicates, when used for cattle and externally, the use of tobacco leaves is not only permitted but encouraged. As the Doctrine and Covenants Institute manual reminds us, "tobacco [has a]   place when used as the Lord intended."[45]

---

[39] George Albert Smith, *Conference Report*, April 1918, p. 40.

[40] Prabhat Jha, "21st-Century Hazards of Smoking and Benefits of Cessation in the United States," *The New England Journal of Medicine*, vol. 368, pp. 341-50.

[41] McMaster University, "Global Study Shows All Tobacco Bad For The Heart," ScienceDaily, 18 August 2006.

[42] National Center for Health Statistics, "Health, United States, 1994," U.S. Department of Health and Human Services. 1995.

[43] Ibid.

[44] Anne Charlton, "Medicinal uses of tobacco in history," *Journal of the Royal Society of Medicine*, vol. 97, no. 6 2004, pp. 292-6.

[45] "Section 89, The Word of Wisdom," Doctrine and Covenants Student Manual, 2001, p. 208.

Drugs

The Word of Wisdom does not specifically mention abuse of legal or illegal drugs within the original text. Some may wonder whether or not they are permitted. To this and other questions about any number of substances, President Joseph Fielding Smith said:

> "Such revelation is unnecessary. The Word of Wisdom is a basic law. It points the way and gives us ample instruction in regard to both food and drink, good for the body and also detrimental. If we sincerely follow what is written with the aid of the Spirit of the Lord, we need no further counsel. Thus by keeping the commandments we are promised inspiration and the guidance of the Spirit of the Lord through which **we will know what is good and what is bad for the body, without the Lord presenting us with a detailed list separating the good things from the bad that we may be protected**. We will learn by this faithful observance that the promises of the Lord are fulfilled."[46]

We ought to use righteous judgment in understanding which substances to avoid and which to utilize. Drugs, which are highly addictive and impair agency, should be avoided. Drugs are unnatural and highly powerful substances. Even small doses and usage can create harmful and lasting effects.

Illicit drugs impact us far more than many of us realize. The cost of drug abuse is estimated to exceed 1 trillion dollars annually.[47] To put this into perspective, that is more than the USA's annual national defense spending.[48] The economic

---

[46] Joseph Fielding Smith, *Improvement Era*, February 1956, pp. 78-79, emphasis added.
[47] Indra Cidambi, "Actual Cost of Drug Abuse in U.S. Tops $1 Trillion Annually," Psychology Today, 10 August 2017.
[48] "National Defense Budget Estimates for FY 2020," United States Department of Defense, Office of the Under Secretary of Defense (Comptroller), May 2019.

implications alone show how illicit drugs have adversely impacted society. In 2018, 67,367 people died of drug overdose in the United States.[49] That is to say nothing of the thousands whose lives have been altered because of drug use, which no report will ever be able to accurately demonstrate. Families are broken apart, jobs are lost, wealth is thrown away, and relationships are forever changed—all for the deceptive and momentary pleasure of these evil substances.

Indeed, abuse of legal and illegal drugs is a plague that has caused untold damage to millions. Surely we would do best to avoid them in any form and keep ourselves far from their addicting power. As President Russel M. Nelson reminds us:

"From trial comes a habit. From habit comes dependence. From dependence comes addiction. Its grasp is so gradual. Enslaving shackles of habit are too small to be sensed until they are too strong to be broken. Indeed, drugs are the modern "mess of pottage" for which souls are sold. No families are free from risk... While we are free to choose, once we have made those choices, we are tied to the consequences of those choices. We are free to take drugs or not. But once we choose to use a habit-forming drug, we are bound to the consequences of that choice. Addiction surrenders later freedom to choose. Through chemical means, one can literally become disconnected from his or her own will!"[50]

Blessings Available to All

So far in this chapter, we have discussed all of the 'don'ts' in the Word of Wisdom and associated health implications from modern research. Of course, the list of things we should avoid putting into our bodies is not limited to what is directly found in

---

[49] Centers for Disease Control and Prevention, "Drug Overdose Deaths," U.S. Department of Health and Human Services, 19 March 2020.
[50] Russell M. Nelson, "Addiction or Freedom," General Conference, October 1988.

the text. The number of substances harmful to the human body created by man will only continue to increase. However, as President Joseph Fielding Smith and many other prophets have taught, the Word of Wisdom is a guiding principle that we should use in conjunction with the Spirit to understand how best to take care of the sacred gift that God has given to each of us— our mortal body.

In our business, we have worked with many members and non-members alike. Most members of the Church we work with already adhere to the list of 'Don'ts.' However, most non-members do not. We work with and counsel these people to cut these harmful substances out of their diets, and when they do, they obtain the associated blessings as well! Indeed, the blessings of the Word of Wisdom are available to all who will abide its principles. However, in order to obtain the full blessings promised by the Lord, it is not enough to simply abstain from harmful substances—else why would He include any additional instruction? There is much more to the Word of Wisdom that we will discuss over the next few chapters.

Chapter Five

The 'Sometimes'

*"And these hath God made for the use
of man only in times of famine and
excess of hunger."*
Doctrine and Covenants 89:15

The Snakes of Zion's Camp

During the summer of 1834, Zion was in turmoil. The Saints
in Missouri had been driven from their lands, and the Lord
commanded that Joseph Smith lead a group of saints from
Kirtland to redeem Zion "by power."[1] What commenced was a
march to Jackson County, Missouri commonly referred to as
Zion's Camp. Along the way, these Saints endured many
hardships and trials. One day as the Prophet was pitching his
tent, the brethren found three prairie rattlesnakes and were
about to kill them. However, Joseph intervened and said:

> "Let them alone—don't hurt them! How will the serpent
> ever lose his venom, while the servants of God possess
> the same disposition, and continue to make war upon it?
> Men must become harmless, before the brute creation;
> and when men lose their vicious dispositions and cease
> to destroy the animal race, the lion and the lamb can
> dwell together, and the sucking child can play with the
> serpent in safety."[2]

---

[1] Doctrine and Covenants 103:15,35.
[2] Joseph Smith, *History of the Church*, vol. 2, p. 71.

Heeding Joseph's words, the brethren carefully picked up the snakes and moved them out of the way. Joseph then went on and "exhorted the brethren not to kill a serpent, bird, or an animal of any kind during our journey unless it became necessary in order **to preserve ourselves from hunger.**"[3] On the surface, this seems like a natural thing for the Lord's prophet to do. However, Joseph records that he taught this principle frequently throughout the travails of Zion's Camp–a principle that is explicitly contained within the Word of Wisdom but is seldom discussed today.

The Most Controversial Portion of the Word of Wisdom

Most faithful members of the Church can agree on a good portion of the Word of Wisdom. We generally know what things we should avoid and what things are good for our bodies. But there is a whole section of the text we rarely, if ever, discuss–the 'sometimes' of the Word of Wisdom. Each time we speak to groups about the Word of Wisdom, there is an awkward tension that quickly permeates the room when we get to the 'sometimes' section. This awkward topic we're referring to is the flesh of beasts and fowls. Indeed, in our day, whenever anyone brings up the topic of eating meat, all kinds of defenses go up about nutritional needs and not being "too extreme." And then, when one suggests that perhaps there is a moral or religious component to refraining from eating animals, people often entrench themselves in their views even more.

This is, perhaps, the most difficult concept about health and the Word of Wisdom to accept; it was for us. So don't put down the book if you do not immediately agree with the information contained in this chapter. Because this information typically cuts against some of our modern preferences, this chapter will contain far more quotes and sources than the other chapters, simply because we want to present the abundance of evidence to

---

[3] Ibid, emphasis added.

you easily and thoroughly. We only ask, as with all sections in this book, that you read with pure intent, compare it with the scriptures, and then take it to the Lord to discover the truth. If anything seems amiss, we would advise you to check it against the scriptures and the words of the prophets. However, that's where we will be drawing all of our support, so buckle up. In fact, many people are surprised to learn that a majority of prophets have made mention about the interpretation of meat consumption in the Word of Wisdom throughout the history of the Church. So, with this in mind, let us begin by examining the text of Section 89 itself.

Sparing God's Creatures

To understand what the Lord expects of us in regards to the consumption of His creations, we turn to verse twelve of Section 89. It reads:

> "Yea, flesh also of beasts and of the fowls of the air, I, the Lord, have ordained for the use of man with thanksgiving; nevertheless **they are to be used sparingly**;"[4]

Often when we discuss our use of meat we stop at saying that it should be used sparingly. This word has numerous meanings to different members. Some believe it means once a meal, others believe it means once a week. Yet others believe that it means just having gratitude when you eat meat. According to one gospel scholar, it simply means sparing God's creatures.[5] Similarly, if we were to employ the aid of the first edition of the Webster's Dictionary published in 1828, sparingly would be defined as "not abundantly," "frugally," "abstinently," "seldom," and "cautiously."[6] From these definitions, we can get a pretty

---

[4] Doctrine and Covenants 89:12, emphasis added.
[5] Hugh Nibley, "The Word of Wisdom: A Commentary on D&C 89," December 1979.
[6] Noah Webster, "sparingly," *An American Dictionary of the English Language*, 1828.

good idea of what this passage meant in the time it was given. However, interpretations aside, we often miss the very next verse where the Lord continues the thought and defines what He means by sparingly:

"And it is pleasing unto me that they **should not be used, only in times of winter, or of cold, or famine.**"[7]

We will never forget the first time that we sat down together to study the Word of Wisdom and this verse hit us over our heads like a ton of bricks. The Lord says here it is pleasing to him that it should NOT be used except in certain situations—those situations being winter, cold, or famine. So, our default should be to not use meat in any capacity, unless we find ourselves in one of the situations described. To us, this was revolutionary. Both of us had taught the Word of Wisdom to investigators on our missions and had no idea these verses existed. These verses are as plain as day within the revelation itself, but when we're not looking for them, we typically roll right past them. However, as we later discovered, latter-day prophets such as Lorenzo Snow have taught this principle plainly and consistently: "Unless famine or extreme cold is upon us we should refrain from the use of meat."[8]

The Lord believed that this information was so important, He put it in the revelation twice. In verse 15 we read, "And these [beasts and fowls] hath God made for the use of man **only in times of famine and excess of hunger.**"[9] Again, the Lord reiterates that only when it is absolutely needful should we turn to the consuming of animal flesh. Now, some may argue that this verse is referring to grains because in verse 14, the Lord talks about grain and its use for man and beast. However, this

---

[7] Doctrine and Covenants 89:13, emphasis added.
[8] Dennis B. Horne, ed., *An Apostle's Record: The Journals of Abraham H. Cannon,* (Clearfield, UT: Gnolaum Books, 2004) p. 424.
[9] Doctrine and Covenants 89:15, emphasis added.

interpretation doesn't make sense, as the footnote on the word "these" in verse 15 directs the reader back to verse 13 where the Lord refers to the use of animal flesh. Perhaps then Elder Joseph Fielding Smith summarized it best:

> "Neither is it the intent of this revelation to include grains and fruits in the restriction placed upon meats, that they should be used only in famine or excess of hunger. The antecedent of "these" in verse 15, may not be clear, but common sense teaches us that it does not refer to grain in the preceding verse."[10]

Many of the early Church brethren taught this principle plainly and consistently. For example, the first recorded talk entirely dedicated to the Word of Wisdom was in the 1842 General Conference. Hyrum Smith, brother of the prophet Joseph Smith and Church Patriarch, spoke in-depth on the blessings, promises, and commands in the Word of Wisdom, giving the most beautiful sermon. He exclaimed:

> "Let men attend to these instructions, let them use the things ordained of God; **let them be sparing of the life of animals; it is pleasing saith the Lord that flesh be used only in times of winter, or of famine.**"[11]

Hyrum was not the only one to talk about this principle. Time and again the brethren emphasized and reiterated the specific times in which we should eat meat; namely winter, cold, and famine. They have made it very clear that the Lord has commanded it to be eaten only in select circumstances and at no other time. In 1857, Heber C. Kimball reminded the Saints that:

---

[10] Joseph Fielding Smith, *Church History and Modern Revelation*, (n.p.: Council of the Twelve Apostles of The Church of Jesus Christ of Latter-day Saints, 1947-1950).
[11] "The Word of Wisdom," *Times and Seasons,* vol. 3, no. 15, p. 801, emphasis added.

> "It is not pleasing in [God's] sight for man to shed blood of beasts. . . **except in times of excess of hunger and famine**. Go and read it for yourselves. . . **It is not the Spirit of God that leads a man or woman to shed blood—to desire to kill and slay**."[12]

These brethren make it very clear that while the flesh of animals is certainly not prohibited, it is meant to be used only in select circumstances.

In the Beginning

To truly understand this concept of sparing God's creatures, we need to go back to the creation of the world. When God created Adam and Eve, the first thing He said to them was to multiply and replenish the earth, with the directive to "subdue it, and have dominion over the fish of the sea, and over the fowl of the air, and over every living thing that moveth upon the earth."[13] The next thing that the Lord did was to tell Adam and Eve exactly what they should eat. In the Genesis account we read:

> "And God said, Behold, I have given you every herb bearing seed, which is upon the face of all the earth, and every tree, in the which is the fruit of a tree yielding seed; **to you it shall be for meat**."[14]

As briefly mentioned in a previous chapter, the instruction given to Adam and Eve was to eat fruit as their primary source of sustenance, as the word 'meat' in Biblical language meant "food in general."[15] Thus it can also be inferred, that this is what is referred to whenever the scriptures use the word 'meat.' When referring to animals, the scriptures typically use the word

---

[12] Heber C. Kimball, *Journal of Discourses*, vol. 6, p. 50, emphasis added.
[13] Genesis 1:28; Moses 2:28.
[14] Genesis 1:29, emphasis added; see also Moses 2:29, Abraham 4:29.
[15] Noah Webster, "meat," *An American Dictionary of the English Language*, 1828.

'flesh.'[16] This instruction to Adam and Eve makes sense considering that the Lord gave it to them before the fall–before death entered the world. From the scriptures, it appears that this instruction remained in force up until the days of Noah, where, in Genesis 9, the Lord gives additional instruction.

After the waters of the Great Flood receded and Noah and his posterity began to dwell on the earth again, the Lord reiterated the command given to Adam and Eve to multiply and replenish the earth. This time, however, the Lord declared in verse 3, "Every moving thing that liveth shall be meat for you; even as the green herb have I given you all things."[17] This is the first instance we have in the scriptures where the Lord sanctions the consumption of animals. But when we read the very next two verses, it gets very confusing. This is because there is a Joseph Smith Translation beginning in verse 4 which reads:

"But, the blood of all flesh which I have given you for meat, shall be shed upon the ground, which taketh life thereof, and the blood ye shall not eat.

And surely, blood shall not be shed, **only for meat, to save your lives**; and **the blood of every beast will I require at your hands**."[18]

From these verses, it appears that the Lord gave Noah the same instruction regarding His creations that we find in the Word of Wisdom–that is, there are only certain times when it is sanctioned to eat them. However, the Lord told Noah that He would require the blood of every beast at Noah's hands if they were slain unnecessarily.

This same sentiment is expressed again in the Doctrine and Covenants when the Lord said, "Wo be unto man that sheddeth

---

[16] Ibid, see "flesh."
[17] Genesis 9:3.
[18] JST Genesis 9:10–11, emphasis added.

blood or that wasteth flesh and **hath no need**."[19] The Lord does not want his children to kill animals for food unless it is absolutely necessary. Surely this cuts against the grain of our modern culture where some form of meat is often the centerpiece of each meal. But when we think about it, all animals are God's creatures and have spirits of their own.[20] Though they have spirits, we also know that they are a lower creation. Man was given dominion or stewardship over animals; we are the higher form of life. We ought to treat all within our influence with love and care. True, the Lord may allow us to take the lives of these lower creations for ours in times of need. Thus, it makes sense that they are for our use, but only when necessary.

Our Stewardship

From the scriptures, we know that God created all living things, including animals, which were created spiritually first, just as we were.[21] However, as God's highest form of creation, humans have dominion over the whole earth. Righteous dominion includes proper care of animals. Animals have the right to life which mankind should respect, as we have been taught by general authorities.[22] Indeed, many prophets and apostles have reminded us that we have an obligation as Latter-day Saints to be kind to animals.[23] As Joseph F. Smith once wrote, "Kindness to the whole animal creation and especially to all domestic animals is not only a virtue that should be developed, but is the absolute duty of mankind."[24]

In addition to teaching kindness towards the animal race, the Prophet Joseph Smith also taught the salvation of animals. He remarked that the animals that John the Revelator saw in vision

---

[19] Doctrine and Covenants 49:21, emphasis added.
[20] Genesis 7:21-22.
[21] Moses 3:5.
[22] George Q. Cannon, "Editorial Thoughts," *Juvenile Instructor,* vol. 9, no. 25, December 1874, p. 294.
[23] David O. McKay, *Conference Report,* October 1951, p. 180.
[24] Joseph F. Smith, "Kindness to Animals," Juvenile Instructor, vol. 47, no. 2, February 1912, p. 79.

were "the most noble animals that had filled the measure of their creation, and had been saved from other worlds, because they were perfect: they were like angels in their sphere."[25] It was clear that Joseph understood this sacred responsibility. Because animals have some form of salvation and have been placed in our care by a loving Heavenly Father, we ought not to take this trust lightly. It is our responsibility to ensure that we follow the Lord's instructions on the matter because to Him, life is sacred. If the Word of Wisdom is a set of principles, then the underlying doctrine of this particular principle would be "Thou shalt not kill."

Other Prophets Agree

On another occasion, Joseph F. Smith spoke of the implications that killing animals can have on our spirit. He said:

> "The unnecessary destruction of life **begets a spirit of destruction which grows within the soul**. It lives by what it feeds upon and robs man of the love that he should have for the works of God. Men cannot worship the Creator and look with careless indifference upon his creation."[26]

President Ezra Taft Benson also warned against the indiscriminate killing of innocent animals.[27] It seems that many prophets saw a correlation between killing an animal and a general hardening of the spirit. Many have agreed and taught about "how dreadful a sin it is to take life. The lives of animals even should be held far more sacred than they are."[28]

Our stewardship and responsibility to take care of these animals is more than just goodwill. We will one day stand

---

[25] Joseph Smith, *History of the Church*, vol. 5, pp. 343-44.
[26] Joseph F. Smith, *Juvenile Instructor*, vol. 53, no. 4, April 1918, pp. 182-3, emphasis added.
[27] Ezra Taft Benson, "A Principle with a Promise," General Conference, April 1983.
[28] George Q. Cannon, *Juvenile Instructor*, vol. 31, no. 7, April 1896, p. 218.

accountable before God for our stewardships, including our treatment of God's animal creations.[29] That day of judgment will not be pleasant if we fail to treat His animals kindly. In fact, as Lorenzo Snow taught:

> "We have no right to slay animals or fowls except from necessity, for **they have spirits which may some day rise up and accuse or condemn us.**"[30]

What we have shown so far should be enough to reexamine our use of animal flesh and even end our overindulgence of meat products. But to ensure that the Saints of these last days understand just how important this directive given in the Word of Wisdom is for our spiritual well being and our health, we will continue with the evidence in support of this idea.

More Reasons to Spare

Many of the Brethren have directly asked us to refrain from eating animals, except in the times provided by the Lord. They have also taught that it is not only unwise, but a sin to kill when there is no need. On the matter, Hyrum Smith remarked, "To kill, when not necessary, is a sin akin to murder."[31] For most of us, when we eat a hamburger or other meat product, we are not going out and shooting the animal ourselves. However, this does not absolve us from any responsibility.

On the same subject, President Lorenzo Snow simply said that "the killing of animals when unnecessary [i]s wrong and sinful."[32] He went on to say that it is not right to focus too much on one aspect of the Word of Wisdom while neglecting other just as important parts.[33] Notice how both teachings echo the idea

---

[29] Doctrine and Covenants 70:4.
[30] Dennis B. Horne, ed., *An Apostle's Record: The Journals of Abraham H. Cannon,* (Clearfield, UT: Gnolaum Books, 2004) p. 424.
[31] Hyrum M. Smith and Janne M. Sjodahl, *Doctrine and Covenants Commentary,* 1919, p. 286.
[32] Historical Department journal history of the Church, 1830-2008; 1890-1899; 5 1898 May, Church History Library.
[33] Ibid.

that meat consumption is only sinful when used unnecessarily. There is a time and a place for animal flesh in our diet, but when we use it outside the bounds the Lord has set it is a sin.

It is clear that the early Presidents and apostles of the Church had strong feelings on the matter and did not mince words (or meat). Their admonitions ought to be enough to warrant our obedience; however, there are many other benefits aside from obedience and the associated blessings. During one General Conference address, George Q. Cannon reminded the Saints that "flesh is not suitable for man in the summer time, and ought to be eaten sparingly in the winter."[34] He also went on to say that other foods could be raised cheaper, in greater variety, and would not take as much preparation time.[35] Here, he taught that our money could be better used on other foods.

What many do not consider is the high cost of meat. Meat is a very expensive form of protein. The average cost of one pound of ground beef in 2019 America is roughly five dollars. By comparison, the average cost of one pound of lentils is one dollar–less than one-fifth the total cost of beef. Nutritionally, the profiles of lentils and ground beef are very similar, except lentils are higher in nutrients and lower in cholesterol. This striking example shows how plant foods are not only cheaper, but more nutritious. Economically speaking, flesh foods are an unwise choice and, as one apostle noted, members of the Church should never complain of scarcity or high price of animal foods.[36]

We are not only told that we are to partake of meat when absolutely necessary, but we are also told that we will be held responsible for the lives that we take when we are not in need. For the glutton who feasts upon meat daily (like we did), that day of reckoning would be quite overwhelming. Luckily for us, the Savior has provided the Atonement. Because of His mercy,

---

[34] George Q. Cannon, *Journal of Discourses*, vol. 12, pp. 221-226.
[35] Ibid.
[36] Joseph F. Merrill, *Conference Report*, April 1948, p. 75.

the transgressions we have committed in ignorance or because of the weakness of our flesh can be wiped clean. That means, for those of us who have struggled with obeying this principle, if we turn our hearts to the Lord in true repentance and utilize the Atonement, we can avoid the testimony of these animals crying against us at the judgment bar of God. By obeying the limits the Lord has set forth, and only eating meat in times of winter, cold or famine, we may have access to the incredible blessings the Lord has promised to the obedient.

What About Forbidding to Abstain?

Perhaps the most common argument raised against this interpretation comes from the Doctrine and Covenants itself. Section 49:18 reads: "And whoso forbiddeth to abstain from meats, that man should not eat the same, is not ordained of God[.]" Many people believe that here the Lord says that if you forbid someone to eat meat, it is not of God. The implication is that a literal reading of God's instruction concerning the flesh of beasts in Section 89 is incorrect. However, this argument does not stand scrutiny.

The idea that one verse would be enough evidence to overturn a multitude of other scriptures and prophetic quotes is rather weak. What we should look for instead is how this verse can work *together* with other scripture and prophetic teachings that appear to be contradictory. This can reasonably be done by turning to the definitions found in the Webster 1828 Dictionary. The word 'forbiddeth' is pretty straightforward and meant "to prohibit;"[37] the word 'abstain' meant "to forbear, or refrain from, voluntarily,"[38] and finally the word 'meat' meant "food in general; any thing eaten for nourishment."[39] When we compile these definitions, the phrase "forbiddeth to abstain from meats" could be re-written in our modern English to read: "whoever

---

[37] Noah Webster, "forbid," *An American Dictionary of the English Language,* 1828.
[38] Ibid, see "abstain."
[39] Ibid, see "meat."

prohibits someone to voluntarily refrain from any food." With this interpretation in mind, the verse would suggest that anyone who prohibits another person from refraining from a food of their own free will and choice is not of God.

There is yet another interpretation of this verse from Dr. Loren Spendlove. He makes the compelling case that the phrase "forbiddeth to abstain" was an idiom of the time—that is, a phrase that is not meant to be understood literally. For example, if we were to say that the Word of Wisdom helped us become "fit as a fiddle," it would be a phrase used to underscore our good health—not a literal commentary on how we look in relation to fiddles. In a similar fashion, Dr. Spendlove shows that this idiom in Section 49 meant "commandeth to abstain."[40] If we swap this phrase into the verse, it would read: "Whoso *commandeth* to abstain from meats, that man should not eat the same. . ." The footnote on 'forbiddeth' appears to confirm this assertion by Dr. Spendlove by suggesting the phrase could read "biddeth to abstain." In this interpretation, the Lord would be saying that anyone who commands another person to abstain from a certain food, particularly meat, that action is not sanctioned by Him.

Does this mean that we *shouldn't* refrain from eating meat? Of course not. The verse is simply saying that if you command someone or force them not to eat meat, that is not of God. This is because God gave them for the use of man as explained in the very next verse: "For, behold, the beasts of the field and the fowls of the air, and that which cometh of the earth, is ordained for the use of man for food and for raiment, and that he might have in abundance."[41] What many people miss, however, is that in verse 21, the Lord reminds His Saints about the sanctity of life by saying: "And wo be unto man that sheddeth blood or that wasteth flesh **and hath no need**."[42] This is consistent with the

---

[40] Loren Spendlove, "Whoso Forbiddeth to Abstain from Meats," *Interpreter: A Journal of Latter-day Saint Faith and Scholarship,* vol. 14, 2015, pp. 17-34. See full article for an in-depth analysis of this phrase.
[41] Doctrine and Covenants 49:19.
[42] Doctrine and Covenants 49:21, emphasis added.

Joseph Smith Translation of Genesis 9 and the circumstances given of the Lord for when to use the flesh of beasts. Thus, when properly understood, the concern over D&C 49:18 should be satisfied.

Eating in the Millenium

It is no secret that we live in the last days before our Savior will make his triumphant return. Many of us have felt the urgency to prepare for what lies ahead. Though none can be sure exactly what is coming and when the Lord will return, it is clear that we are not far from this prophesied time. As President Russell M. Nelson remarked in 2016, the "Millennial" generation has a great role to play in the Second Coming and it is very possible that they may be the Lord's Millennial people.[43] Though no man knows the day, nor the hour, some days it feels like we are in the proverbial "week" of the Second Coming and we ought to be prepared.[44] What better way to prepare than by living *all* of God's commands? This surely includes the Word of Wisdom.

Those who will be alive during the Savior's millennial reign will not partake of any meat, just as in the days of Adam. This may come as a shock to some, but the scriptures make this abundantly clear. Isaiah, in prophesying of the Millenium, says that all animals shall lie together and lions shall eat straw. It goes on to say that "none shall hurt nor destroy."[45] These were the verses Joseph Smith referred to when he reprimanded the men of Zion's Camp and admonished them not to harm any animal unless it was to preserve their lives. Clearly, this indicates that no animal blood shall be spilled during the Millennium. This is reiterated in the Doctrine and Covenants which teaches us that in that day there will be no enmity between man and beast.[46] President Lorenzo Snow taught that the Saints violated the use of meat just as much or more than other aspects of the

---

[43] Russell M. Nelson, "Stand as True Millennials," *Ensign*, October 2016.
[44] Matthew 24:36.
[45] Isaiah 11:6-9.
[46] Doctrine and Covenants 101:26.

Word of Wisdom. He went on to say that the time was near when "Latter-day Saints should be taught to refrain from meat-eating and shedding of animal blood."[47]

His words teach us that in a future day, the Church will again teach the people to strictly refrain from meat of any kind. Elder Bruce R. McConkie gave more insight into what the diet of the Millennium might look like for the righteous Saints: "Man and all forms of life will be vegetarians in the coming day; the eating of meat will cease, because, for one thing, death as we know it ceases. There will be no shedding of blood."[48]

Joseph Fielding Smith also weighed in on the matter of the Millennial diet. In a letter, he once wrote:

> "When [the millennium comes] we will learn that the eating of meat is not good for us. Why do we feel that we do not have a square meal unless it is based largely on meat? Let the dumb animals live. They enjoy life as well as we do. . . . Naturally, in times of famine the flesh of animals was perhaps a necessity, but in my judgment when the Millennium reaches us, we will live above the need of killing dumb innocent animals and eating them. If we will take this stand in my judgment, we may live longer."[49]

If that is the proper diet in the Lord's Kingdom upon the earth, wouldn't it stand to reason that it is the proper diet to prepare for His return? We are not fond of the argument that "I might as well live it up now and eat all of my bacon if I don't get any in the Millenium." To those who wish to "Eat, drink and be merry, for tomorrow we die," Nephi responded by reminding us

---

[47] Leonard J. Arrington, "An Economic Interpretation of the 'Word of Wisdom,'" *Brigham Young University Studies*, vol. 1, no. 1, 1959, p. 47.

[48] Bruce R. McConkie, *Millennial Messiah*, (Salt Lake City, UT: Deseret Book Company, 1982), pp. 658-9.

[49] Letter to a member sister in El Paso, Texas, dated 30 Dec. 1966, quoted in *Health Is A Blessing: A Guide to the Scriptural Laws of Good Health*, by Steven H. Horne, (Springville, Utah: Nature's Field, 1994), p. 34.

that this thought process is from the devil.[50] We believe that we are best served preparing for our future estate, whether in heaven or the Millennium, by living these principles now. Since there will be no bloodshed in heaven nor on earth during this time, there will be no meat-eating, either. Although the Lord issues no directive in the Word of Wisdom about living this now, perhaps it would be wise to at least consider these things.

Modern Research Overcomes Nutritional Objections

As we showed, Joseph Fielding Smith estimated that the eating of meat is not good for us and that if we refrained, we would live longer. However, he believed that we wouldn't learn this until the Millennium. He would probably be thrilled to know that it hasn't taken the advent of the Millennium to obtain this knowledge.

Hundreds of studies now confirm what the Lord revealed nearly 200 years ago about our consumption of meat—it is not, in fact, good for our bodies. Before diving into some of this evidence, however, we want to remind the reader that to have faith in and obey revealed principles, we do not need modern science to confirm their efficacy. But it is exciting to note and reassuring to the obedient when man's wisdom catches up with the wisdom of the Lord.

Upon hearing that meat ought not to be regularly consumed, one of the first nutritional concerns is usually about protein intake or, perhaps, sufficient B12 levels. Indeed, many questions are often raised about the health implications of abstaining from meat. What many do not realize is that more data is being released every day showing that our bodies are not only equipped to function without meat, but it is optimal to refrain. There is now a large body of evidence indicating that animal

---

[50] 2 Nephi 28:7-8,21.

foods lead to significant health complications.[51] Those that eat a more plant-based diet can suppress cancer 80 percent more than those on a diet of animal foods.[52] Other studies have found that even "moderate" consumption of meat is devastating to health. One study found that eating meat once a week leads to 146 percent increase in risk of heart disease, 152 percent increase in risk of stroke, 166 percent increase in risk of diabetes, 231 percent increase in risk of weight gain and a 3.6 year decrease in life expectancy.[53]

Concerning B12, it is a bacterium made by anaerobic microorganisms that grow in the dirt.[54] Because of modern farming practices, the bacteria have been depleted to the point that it is nearly impossible for anyone to get adequate B12 without supplementation.[55] That's why studies show that proportionate amounts of omnivores and vegans have a B12 deficiency.[56] It is untrue that those who do not eat meat are B12 deficient at a higher rate than those who are not. It is often argued that animal products contain B12, but this is only because animals are injected with B12 before being slaughtered.[57] Thus, it is easier to skip the middleman (or middle

[51] Michael Greger, *How Not to Die,* (New York, NY: Flatiron Books, 2015), pp. 36-39, 66-70, 107.

[52] Dean Ornish et al., "Intensive lifestyle changes may affect the progression of prostate cancer," *The Journal of urology,* vol. 174, no. 3, 2005, pp. 1065-70.

[53] Pramil N Singh et al., "Global epidemiology of obesity, vegetarian dietary patterns, and noncommunicable disease in Asian Indians," *The American journal of clinical nutrition,* vol. 100 Suppl 1,1, 2014, pp. 359S-64S.

[54] University of Kent, "Scientific breakthrough reveals how vitamin B12 is made," *ScienceDaily,* 8 August 2013.

[55] Thomas Campbell, "12 Questions Answered Regarding Vitamin B12," *Center for Nutrition Studies,* 6 February 2015.

[56] Katherine L. Tucker et al., "Plasma vitamin B-12 concentrations relate to intake source in the Framingham Offspring study," *American Journal of Clinical Nutrition,* vol. 71, no. 2, Feb 2000 pp. 514-22.

[57] C L Girard et al., "Apparent ruminal synthesis and intestinal disappearance of vitamin B12 and its analogs in dairy cows," *Journal of dairy science,* vol. 92, no. 9, 2009, pp. 4524-9.

cow) and supplement directly with a B12 vitamin 1-2x per week, because those who eat meat still have to supplement.[58]

Others are concerned about adequate protein intake. A protein is a combination of 22 amino acids.[59] Some of these amino acids are produced naturally in the body, so we don't have to worry about them. The remaining 9 amino acids are what we call "essential," which means our body does not naturally produce them and they must be supplemented with food. The good news is that these amino acids all originate in dirt and plant foods![60] That means the best way to get these amino acids is from plants. Many are shocked to find that there is virtually no such thing as protein deficiency. Just the opposite is true. A recent study found that a high animal protein intake is associated with a 75 percent increased risk in overall mortality and a 400 percent increase in cancer.[61] In essence, it's more likely that you can have *too much* protein rather than too little.

Surprisingly, our best source of protein comes from plants. It is also important to note that studies indicate our bodies need only about 10 percent of our daily caloric intake to be from protein.[62] That means the average 150 lb. person only needs about 50 grams of protein per day, even for bodybuilders.[63] Furthermore, overconsumption of protein, in particular animal protein, is linked to autoimmune diseases such as diabetes,

---

[58] See Campbell "12 Questions Answered Regarding Vitamin B12."

[59] Neil Osterweil, "The Benefits of Protein," *WebMD*.

[60] John McDougall, "Plant foods have a complete amino acid composition," *Circulation*, vol. 105, no. 25, June 2002, e197.

[61] Morgan E. Levine et al., "Low protein intake is associated with a major reduction in IGF-1, cancer, and overall mortality in the 65 and younger but not older population," *Cell metabolism*, vol. 19, no. 3, 2014, pp. 407-17.

[62] D. Joe Millward, "Identifying recommended dietary allowances for protein and amino acids: a critique of the 2007 WHO/FAO/UNU report," *The British journal of nutrition*, vol. 108, Suppl 2, 2012, pp. S3-21.

[63] Institute of Medicine, *Dietary Reference Intakes: The Essential Guide to Nutrient Requirements*, Washington, DC: The National Academies Press, 2006, pp. 144-6.

kidney disease, MS, IBS, and Lyme disease.[64] One study found a significantly increased risk of developing diabetes on a high animal protein diet.[65] Another study found a 60 percent *increased* risk of heart disease on an animal protein diet and a 40 percent *decreased* risk on a diet of plant-sourced proteins.[66] These studies and many others indicate that plant sources are not only a superior form of protein but they lead to significantly improved health outcomes. From a scholastic perspective, the data is overwhelming. Considering the state of human health in America and among the Church membership, we ought to consider the implications of meat consumption on our souls and our health.

Testimony of the Authors

We realize that for many members this topic can be a sensitive one because of the culture in which we live and the traditions that follow. We understand that much of the language from the scriptures and some Church leaders can feel pretty harsh. We don't expect every person to agree with the evidence presented or even with early Church leaders.   We're also understanding of other common objections raised such as "The Brethren don't eat this way," or "Christ ate fish." To adequately answer these would require a much deeper discussion which falls outside of the scope of this work but will be answered at another time. However, even with these objections in mind, they certainly cannot supersede what is written in scripture and what has been consistently taught by Church authorities. For now, the only thing we can do is invite you to seek revelation on the

[64] Ioannis Delimaris, "Adverse Effects Associated with Protein Intake above the Recommended Dietary Allowance for Adults," *ISRN nutrition,* vol. 2013, July 2013.

[65] InterAct Consortium et al., "Association between dietary meat consumption and incident type 2 diabetes: the EPIC-InterAct study." *Diabetologia,* vol. 56, no. 1, 2013, pp. 47-59.

[66] Marion Tharrey et al., "Patterns of plant and animal protein intake are strongly associated with cardiovascular mortality: the Adventist Health Study-2 cohort," *International Journal of Epidemiology,* vol. 47, no. 5, October 2018, pp. 1603–1612.

matter, because this is what we had to do for ourselves with this very same subject.

Out of all the principles contained within Section 89, this was perhaps the one we violated the most. So while Cassidy was frustrated with the relentless sickness and pain, she had no claim on the promised blessings because she was not living it exactly. We always believed Jordan to be the healthier of either of us, but, as we mentioned previously, one doctor's test showed that he had early warning signs of heart disease (one of the symptoms of eating too much meat), even though he was only a thin 23-year-old! Knowing what we know now, this shouldn't have come as a surprise because we had some form of meat at every single meal. Many hundreds of animals were killed for our enjoyment.

When we discovered that it might be a violation of the Word of Wisdom to unnecessarily eat animals, we rejected the notion and made excuses and rationalized our behavior. However, we were soon convinced through the whisperings of the Holy Ghost that we had to change not only for our health but for our spirits as well. How grateful we are for the Lord and His mercy, who extends the arm of forgiveness when we realize we have done wrong and seek to make amends! We had neglected the stewardship and responsibility He set upon us through our ancestors, but now we committed to do better.

We decided to give up meat and all other animal foods except in the circumstances outlined by the Lord for a two-week trial. Today, we joke that we are still in that trial. It is because of this change that both of us were able to feel the "health in [our] navel[s] and marrow in [our] bones" and to "run and not be weary."[67] After several months of this "experiment," Jordan's blood work came back clean—no signs of heart disease whatsoever. Cassidy's blood work also showed no signs of inflammation or any of the diseases that previously afflicted her

---

[67] Doctrine and Covenants 89:18,20.

body. Even more important than what the test results showed, however, was that the constant stomach pains were no more; the migraines had subsided; the achy joints soothed, and the once-chronic kidney stones never returned!

While our health has been an absolute gift that we cherish dearly, perhaps the most important blessing we have experienced since making this change has been a greater abundance of the Holy Ghost in our lives. When we are responsible for the death of life (directly or indirectly), as President Joseph F. Smith taught, a spirit of destruction enters into our hearts, and we put ourselves at odds with God. In this state, it can be hard to hear the soft whisperings of the Spirit. When we cleared our minds and spirits of this dark cloud, we began to realize the promise made in the Word of Wisdom that those who keep it would "find wisdom and great treasures of knowledge, even hidden treasures."[68] Indeed, since the time that we made a better effort to follow the whole of the Word of Wisdom, we have seen things in the scriptures we didn't see before and we have had precious revelations from the Lord for the edification of our family. We can say with confidence that had we not followed this principle, these things would not have happened.

Our experience is certainly not unique. There are many Saints in our day who have similar stories and experiences. What we the authors have noticed in recent years, however, is an increasing number of people who feel like they need to live the Word of Wisdom better but aren't sure how or why. Hopefully, this chapter will serve as a "next step" for many people wanting to live the Word of Wisdom more fully. However, just as important as what we don't put into our body (if not more) is what we *do* put into our body, which we will cover in the next chapter.

---

[68] Doctrine and Covenants 89:19.

Chapter Six

The 'Dos'

*"Prove thy servants, I beseech thee,
ten days; and let them give us pulse to
eat, and water to drink."*
Daniel 1:12

The Daniel Diet

Around 597 B.C., Babylonian King Nebuchadnezzar besieged
and captured Jerusalem. As a result, he took many of the Jews
back to Babylon as captives. Included in this group were the
"best and brightest" in Israel.[1] The idea was to teach and train
these bright young ones and make them into Babylonians.
Among those of the best and brightest were Daniel, Hananiah,
Mishael, and Azariah.[2] Part of their training was to be fed a rich
diet of "kingly food" which would have certainly included large
quantities of meat, wine, expensive cheeses, etc. Daniel, as the
leader of these righteous boys, rejected these foods and "would
not defile himself with the portion of the king's meat, nor with
the wine which [the king] drank."[3] In their new Babylonian
home, this unthinkable act was likely to get all four of them
killed. Yet, Daniel insisted that he would not defile himself.
Instead, this brave young man petitioned that they be fed a diet
of pulse and water.[4] Some may ask, what is pulse? According to

---

[1] Daniel 1:4.
[2] Daniel 1:6.
[3] Daniel 1:8.
[4] Daniel 1:12.

the 1828 Webster Dictionary, pulse meant a combination of beans, peas, seeds, or legumes.[5] In other words, Daniel asked for a carb-loaded vegetable, bean, and seed dish for every meal. He knew that this was life or death and he needed to get stronger and healthier faster than his peers. With the stakes so high, why would he choose plant foods to accomplish this goal?

The chief official was not pleased with this proposition and was uninterested in granting exceptions. However, a lesser steward was sympathetic to their plight and reluctantly complied by granting them a 10-day test of this seemingly inferior diet.[6] After the trial period, these Israelite boys were compared against their meat-eating, wine-drinking counterparts, and the diet of pulse was the clear victor! Daniel and his friends, according to Daniel's account, were stronger and fairer in appearance.[7] The results were so incredible after just 10 days, that the chief official quickly changed the diet of each of the other boys to a diet of pulse.[8]

This incredible story is often discussed in conjunction with the Word of Wisdom, but rarely is it used to exemplify the ideal diet. Why would Daniel reject the meat offered to him? Is it because he understood just how good plant foods are for the body? Perhaps he understood the 'Dos' of the Word of Wisdom thousands of years before the revelation we know was even revealed.

Too often we focus on the 'Don'ts' of the Word of Wisdom but rarely do we realize that there are more verses dedicated to admonitions than prohibitions. When we ignore the things that we have been commanded to use, we are missing out on a big part of the Word of Wisdom. As Lorenzo Snow reminded us, it is "not right to neglect part of the Word of Wisdom and be too

---

[5] Noah Webster, "pulse," *An American Dictionary of the English Language*, 1828.
[6] Daniel 1:14.
[7] Daniel 1:15.
[8] Daniel 1:16.

strenuous in regard to other parts."[9]   In other words, what we put into our bodies is just as important as what we *do not* put into our bodies. We have spoken with many faithful Saints who would never drink coffee or alcohol, but who reject the Lord's counsel that grains should be the staff of our lives. Doctrine and Covenants 89 identifies a list of items that are suitable for us to eat. Grains, herbs, and fruit are singled out and specifically mentioned in the text and should, therefore, be a primary focus of our diet. While unsurprising to men like Daniel, it sometimes comes as a shock to Latter-day Saints that the Lord has counseled us to eat primarily carbohydrates. In this chapter, we will discuss in-depth the Lord's counsel to us on the proper diet and how we can better utilize these foods.

Herbs and Their General Use

In the Word of Wisdom, the Lord lays out very specifically what things are good for our food and what should be used. He says:

> "And again, verily I say unto you, all wholesome herbs God hath ordained for the **constitution, nature and use of man**. Every herb **in the season** thereof, and every fruit in the season thereof all these to be used with prudence and thanksgiving. . . All grain is good for the food of man; as also the fruit of the vine; that which yieldeth fruit, whether in the ground or above the ground."[10]

To better help us understand what the implications of these verses are, let us look at a few definitions from the 1828 American Dictionary of the English Language by Noah Webster. These definitions will help to better understand the intent

---

[9] Historical Department journal history of the Church, 1830-2008; 1890-1899; 1898 May, Church History Library.
[10] Doctrine and Covenants 89:10-11;16, emphasis added.

behind each phrase and allow us to gain a more complete picture of what the Lord intended in the revelation.

First, herbs are singled out for us, specifically for our constitution, nature, and use. Does this mean we should be eating a diet of oregano and rosemary? While this may be what comes to mind when we hear the word herbs, the 1828 dictionary offers much greater insight:

> HERB – A plant or vegetable with a soft or succulent stalk or stem, which dies to the root every year, and is thus distinguished from a tree and a shrub.[11]

In this definition, we learn that herbs encompass almost every plant that is edible. The Lord also adds that this includes every fruit above ground or below ground, which would include trees. The insight from this definition means that this revelation is not only talking about oregano and rosemary (although we will discuss those kinds of herbs in the next chapter), but also encompasses beans, nuts, seeds, dark leafy greens, tubers, fruits, vegetables, and more. To go another step further, let's look at the Webster definitions for constitution, nature, and use to determine how the Lord wants us to use them.

> CONSTITUTION – The state of being; that form of being or peculiar structure and connection of parts which makes or characterizes a system or body. Hence the particular frame or temperament of the human body is called its constitution.[12]

> NATURE – The essence, essential qualities or attributes of a thing, which constitute it what it is. When we speak of the nature of man, we understand the peculiar

---

[11] Noah Webster, "herb," *An American Dictionary of the English Language,* 1828.
[12] Ibid, see "constitution."

constitution of his body or mind, or the qualities of the species which distinguish him from other animals.[13]

USE – The act of handling or employing in any manner, and for any purpose, but especially for a profitable purpose.[14]

We need to understand exactly what the Lord means here. According to the above definitions, plant foods are to be a central part in regulating the frame and temperament of our bodies. They are also to be an essential part of our lives and can be handled by us for any purpose. What broad definitions with so many applications! The Lord is essentially telling us that if it grows in nature, we can and should focus on it as a primary element of our diet, health regimen, and whatever other purposes we can conceive. Additionally, because foods such as fruits, vegetables, herbs, and grains are singled out here, one can conclude that any fad, diet, or professional advocating to limit them is not in line with what our Creator has declared.

The scriptural evidence for this view is abundant. The Lord continually singles out these plant foods as the primary source of food for His children. In all three creation accounts in Latter-day Saint scripture, the Lord tells Adam and Eve that plant foods should be their primary source of food. The Genesis account reads:

> "And God said, Behold, I have given you **every herb bearing seed**, which is upon the face of all the earth, and every tree, in the which is the fruit of a tree yielding seed; **to you it shall be for meat** (food)."[15]

God intended these herbs or plants to be our main source of food because, as many authorities have pointed out, when the Lord uses "shall" language, He is saying it is a commandment.

---

[13] Ibid, see "nature."
[14] Ibid, see "use."
[15] Genesis 1:29.

Therefore, we can conclude that the Lord *commanded* Adam and Eve to eat plants. Orson Pratt also felt this was the case. He argued that men and women, starting from the time of Adam and Eve, were made to eat fruits and vegetables. He says:

> "For it will be remembered that animals did not devour one another until after the fall, neither was there any death, until after the fall. What did they eat, then? The Lord said, 'To every beast of the field, and to every thing that creepeth upon the earth, wherein there is life, I have given every green herb for meat.' **The grass, and the herbs, and every green thing were their food**. And Adam and Eve ate fruits and vegetables, not animal flesh."[16]

This sentiment is echoed all over in scripture. From Psalms[17] to the Book of Mormon.[18] As President Gordon B. Hinckley indicated, God is pleased when we eat these foods and it saddens Him that we do not obey this admonition more faithfully.[19] As a Saint, pleasing God ought to be our top priority. As such, we would be wise to eat the foods that please Him and avoid the foods which do not.

Prophets old and new have consistently admonished God's people to eat a diet composed of fruits and vegetables. Daniel denied the "king's meat" for a diet of pulse.[20] President Brigham Young may be the prophet with the most recorded opinions on diet and nutrition. During a long life plagued with disease, he felt that a proper diet did more for his health than the doctor. President Young simply stated that "When men live to the age of a tree, their food will be fruit."[21] On other occasions, he scolded

---

[16] Orson Pratt, *Journal of Discourses,* vol. 20, p. 18, emphasis added.
[17] Psalm 104:14.
[18] Alma 46:40.
[19] Gordon B. Hinckley, "Mormon Should Mean 'More Good'," General Conference, October 1990.
[20] Daniel 1:8.
[21] Brigham Young, *Journal of Discourses,* vol. 8, p. 63.

Saints for eating unhealthy foods that did not feed the body and make room for the Spirit.[22] Even then President of the Quorum of the Twelve Ezra Taft Benson taught that we need to put more focus on fruits, vegetables, and grains. He went on to say:

> "To a significant degree, we are an overfed and undernourished nation digging an early grave with our teeth, and lacking the energy that could be ours because we overindulge in junk foods. . . .**we need a generation of young people who, as Daniel, eat in a more healthy manner than to fare on the 'king's meat' — and whose countenances show it.**"[23]

The prophets have understood the incredible blessings to be gained by following these admonitions in the Word of Wisdom and from the example of Daniel. Not only have the prophets emphasized that fruits and vegetables should be the center of our diet, but the Lord Himself has as well. In addition to these, the Lord has also specified that grain should play a major role.

Grain

In verses 14-17 of the Word of Wisdom the Lord advises on the use of grains. He says:

> "All grain is ordained for the use of man and of beasts, **to be the staff of life ... All grain is good for the food of man**; as also the fruit of the vine; that which yieldeth fruit, whether in the ground or above the ground."[24]

That series of verses ought to be enough to shock a Keto dieter right out of Ketosis! It sure shocked us! The Lord identifies here that grains should be a primary source of calories for all of His Saints. Grains are meant to be the staff of life or, in

[22] John. A. Widtsoe, *Discourses of Brigham Young*, (Salt Lake City, UT: Deseret Book Company, 1951), p. 189.
[23] Ezra Taft Benson, *Teachings of Ezra Taft Benson*, (Salt Lake City, UT: Bookcraft, 1988), p. 476-77, emphasis added.
[24] Doctrine and Covenants 89:14-17, emphasis added.

other words, a staple in our diet. Again, this is consistent with the Biblical counsel the Lord gave Adam and Eve when He said it was by the sweat of their brows that they would eat bread.[25]

In the Book of Mormon, there are over 25 mentions of grain. Studying each of these passages reveals an interesting theme. When the Nephites were obedient to God they were described as being prosperous, and in many cases, it is also mentioned that they raised grain abundantly.[26] The use of grains throughout the Book of Mormon is associated with obedience and a flourishing society.[27] On the other hand, when the Lamanites were disobedient and idolatrous, they are described as being "blood thirsty."[28] Enos even goes as far as to say that they were evil because they fed on the beasts of prey.[29] An interesting juxtaposition for us to consider the relationship of righteousness and the foods we eat. God's people have always had grains as a staple of their diet, so why would now be any different?

This may seem confusing, given the fact that we spent an entire section in the Conspiring Men chapter exposing the secret combinations that have manipulated and altered wheat. However, that conspiring men would put so much effort into changing wheat only confirms that it must be important. Unfortunately, those that aren't exploiting wheat are often advocating against its use entirely. As such, diet trends like the Paleo and Keto diets, which exclude grains entirely, have risen in popularity over the last five years.[30] These diets, which are exciting because of their quick results, appear to be the opposite of what the Lord has advised. Is it any wonder the Lord said that the Word of Wisdom was for all Saints in the last days? Surely,

---

[25] Moses 4:25.
[26] Helaman 6:12.
[27] Alma 1:29.
[28] Mosiah 10:12.
[29] Enos 1:20.
[30] Kristiana Lalou, "Diet trends of 2020: Intermittent fasting and keto in the limelight," Nutrition Insight, 7 January 2020.

He knew of the coming diet trends and gave us a blueprint to avoid all of the confusion.

So, the question remains, if wheat has been so maligned, and the modern wheat product is just a smorgasbord of harmful chemicals that are bad for us, what are we to do? The answer, again, lies in the 1828 Webster Dictionary. According to its definition of wheat, wheat is classified as a plant in the Triticum genus, which includes over 30,000 different strains and varieties![31] Just a few popular examples are spelt, emmer, einkorn, and farro. This means that the two to three strains that we consider "wheat" today are just a handful of types of wheat, leaving over 29,997 remaining strains for our use as well. Some of the other common varieties not already mentioned include grains such as teff, oats, quinoa, buckwheat, rice, amaranth, millet, and sorghum. Looking at other sources of wheat and grain can benefit us greatly. These varieties contain a better nutrient profile and have been far less contaminated by men.[32]

Ultimately, grains can and should be a primary source of food for us. We are told that they should be the staff of life and that all grains are good for the food of man.[33] Some may wonder, if the Lord has ordained *all* grains for our use, why sound the alarm against genetically modified and hybridized grains? Wouldn't those also be included in "all grains?" This is a great question worthy of exploration. Let's think about fruit for a moment—say a peach. Are peaches healthy for you? Yes! No doubt. God perfectly designed a beautiful peach to be full of vitamins, minerals, nutrients, and much more. What about a peach sprayed with herbicides, fungicides, and pesticides that are linked to serious health complications and which also kill the good bacteria beneficial to the human body? What about when

---

[31] Noah Webster, "wheat," An American Dictionary of the English Language, 1828.
[32] Raymond Cooper, "Re-discovering ancient wheat varieties as functional foods," *Journal of Traditional and Complementary Medicine*, vol. 5, no. 3, July 2015, pp. 138-43.
[33] Doctrine and Covenants 89:16.

this same chemically-treated peach is canned with high fructose corn syrup, sugar, colorants, and preservatives? Are these two peaches—the natural and the man-made—equal? It should be obvious to each person that a freshly picked peach is far better for your health than a canned and sugared peach. It is the same with grains. We have taken God's design and we have altered it, changed its composition, and essentially said, "God's way was not good enough. We need man's wisdom to fix it." Ironically, studies have shown that man-made chemicals do not increase crop yields as previously thought.[34] Moreover, these genetically modified foods have an entirely different nutritional profile, with much lower overall nutrition than organically grown foods.[35] Therefore, we can conclude that while all grains are good for our use, we should take great care to ensure that the grains we use have not been perverted by man.

In short, grains are of great importance to us. It is no coincidence that the Lord spends four entire verses in the Word of Wisdom talking about it! We can reasonably conclude that any diet prohibiting or severely restricting grains ought to be rejected, as it does not fall in line with the Word of Wisdom.

Debunking Myths About Carbohydrates

Now that we have established what the Lord has said about what we *should* eat, we will now turn our attention to addressing many secular concerns. In the world today, many people believe that the foods the Lord says are good are not ones we should enjoy. Indeed, the foods the Lord prescribes are largely made up of carbohydrates, and if there is one food group that has been maligned more than any others today, it is carbohydrates. Many are afraid that eating carbohydrates will cause them to gain

---

[34] Doug Gurian-Sherman, "Failure to Yield: Evaluating the Performance of Genetically Engineered Crops," Union of Concerned Scientists, April 2009, pp. 2-4.

[35] T Bøhn et al., "Compositional "differences in soybeans on the market: glyphosate accumulates in Roundup Ready GM soybeans," *Food Chemistry*, vol. 153, 2014, pp. 207-15.

weight, get diabetes, etc. This sad perspective couldn't be farther from the truth. Carbohydrates ought to be our best friends. First, because the Lord makes clear that these are the foods ordained for our use, and second, because modern science has given us a great deal of data to support the use of these carbohydrates in our diet. Though we do not need modern science to confirm what God has taught, it is interesting to note that there are many health benefits to a carbohydrate-centered diet, focusing on fruits and vegetables. All of our needs are met with this kind of diet.

Before we talk about the benefits of these carbohydrates it is important to note *which* carbohydrates we are talking about. A Word of Wisdom sanctioned, carbohydrate-rich diet would consist of foods like tubers, fruits, vegetables, dark leafy greens, grains, seeds, nuts, beans, lentils, etc. We are *not* talking about cake, cookies, donuts, cereal, soda, candy, etc. Those items would be in the category of foods to *avoid* simply because they have been refined and processed to the point where they offer little nutritional value. So as we move forward, keep in mind that the kind of carbohydrates we are discussing are the unadulterated plant foods that Heavenly Father has given for our use, not man-made sugar traps.

Plants are the perfectly crafted foods for our health and wellbeing. They contain every single necessary vitamin, mineral, nutrient, and phytochemical that your body needs to flourish.[36] As Elder John A. Widstoe pointed out in his book on the Word of Wisdom:

> "Plants contain all of the necessary food substances: proteins, fats, starches, and other carbohydrates, minerals and water [and vitamins]. The great Builder of

---

[36] Ben Brown, "Does Ornish Lifestyle Medicine Help with Pre-Diabetes and Diabetes? I Thought I Needed More Protein, Fat and Less Carbs," Ornish Lifestyle Medicine, Ornish.com.

the earth provided well for the physical needs of His children."[37]

Just as Elder Widstoe proclaims, plants are sufficient for our dietary needs. But this is not what the world would have you believe. Low-carbohydrate diets are more popular than ever and even well-educated nutrition professionals would have you believe that carbohydrates lead to bad health. However, carbs are essential to every tissue and cell in our entire body.[38] Our brains, for instance, require carbohydrate-created glucose to function. The brain is unable to function on a diet of fat or protein, exclusively. That is why we hear of Keto Diet "brain fog." The brain is starving, creating immediate and long term repercussions. One study found that after women followed a "low-carbohydrate" diet for just one week, their working memory and visuospatial memory drastically declined.[39] More scary than brain fog, however, is that low-carbohydrate diets are directly associated with early death.[40] Some studies have classified these diets as extremely unsafe and have indicated that they lead to poor long-term health.[41]

Numerous studies have indicated that high-carbohydrate diets have also been found to be the best diet for weight loss and

---

[37] John A. Widtsoe and Leah D. Widtsoe, The Word of Wisdom A Modern Interpretation, (Salt Lake City, UT: Deseret Book Company 1950), p. 127.

[38] Hardy, Karen, et al., "The Importance of Dietary Carbohydrate in Human Evolution," The Quarterly Review of Biology, vol. 90, no. 3, 2015, pp. 251–268.

[39] Kristen E. D'anci et al., "Low-carbohydrate weight-loss diets. Effects on cognition and mood," Appetite, vol. 52, 2009, pp. 96-103.

[40] Sara B. Seidelmann et al., "Dietary carbohydrate intake and mortality: a prospective cohort study and meta-analysis," The Lancet, vol. 3, no. 9, 1 September 2018, pp. E419-28.

[41] "Low carbohydrate diets are unsafe and should be avoided," European Society of Cardiology, 28 August 2018, Press Release.

long-term health.[42] Those who eat the most carbohydrates have the lowest risk for heart disease, type 2 diabetes, and obesity.[43]

Another benefit of carbohydrates is their fiber content. An estimated 97% of the population is fiber deficient and these deficiencies are linked to a host of health problems.[44] Researchers at BYU found that those who increased their fiber intake lost weight and those who ate a low-fiber (low-carbohydrate) diet gained weight.[45] Since fiber is not found in animal proteins or fats and only in carbohydrate foods, we start to see why carbs are so important![46]

Some claim that we should limit our fruit consumption for better health. As we have already discussed, Adam and Eve were commanded to eat fruit. It should stand to reason that fruit should be a primary source of our food as well. Moreover, numerous studies have found a correlation between higher fruit intake and fewer problems with diabetes, heart disease, and many other common health problems of our day.[47] Fruit is not

---

[42] Hana Kahleova et al., "A Plant-Based High-Carbohydrate, Low-Fat Diet in Overweight Individuals in a 16-Week Randomized Clinical Trial: The Role of Carbohydrates," *Nutrients*, vol. 10, no. 9, 2018, p. 1302.

[43] "The Carbohydrate Advantage," *Physicians Committee for Responsible Medicine*, https://www.pcrm.org/good-nutrition/nutrition-information/the-carbohydrate-advantage.

[44] Alanna Moshfegh et al., *What We Eat in America*, NHANES 2001-2002: Usual Nutrient Intakes from Food Compared to Dietary Reference Intakes, U.S. Department of Agriculture, Agricultural Research Service, 2005.

[45] Larry A. Tucker and Kathryn S. Thomas, "Increasing Total Fiber Intake Reduces Risk of Weight and Fat Gains in Women," *The Journal of Nutrition*, vol. 139, no. 3, March 2009, pp. 576-81.

[46] "Understanding Fiber," Diabetes Education Online, *University of California, San Francisco*, https://dtc.ucsf.edu/living-with-diabetes/diet-and-nutrition/understanding-carbohydrates/counting-carbohydrates/learning-to-read-labels/understanding-fiber/

[47] Isao Muraki et al., "Fruit consumption and risk of type 2 diabetes: results from three prospective longitudinal cohort studies." *BMJ (Clinical research ed.)*, vol. 347, 28 Aug. 2013, p. f5001. See also Dagfinn Aune et al,. "Fruit and vegetable intake and the risk of cardiovascular disease, total cancer and all-cause mortality-a systematic review and dose-response meta-analysis of prospective studies." *International journal of epidemiology*, vol. 46, no. 3, 2017, pp. 1029-56.

the culprit of poor health. It is one of the main indicators of good health![48]

Carbohydrates are an amazing source of food for nearly every single person regardless of location or resources. Unrefined carbohydrates such as beans and grains can be found for roughly one-fifth of the total price of animal protein and fat sources, which is lean on the budget as well as your body. They store for long periods, are easy to prepare, and they can be grown with minimal land and effort. There is no one who wouldn't benefit in nearly every aspect by eating more of these kinds of carbs as advised in the Word of Wisdom.

The Ideal Diet

Some may ask, "What is the ideal diet?" To this question, we would answer: the diet that Daniel ate and what the Word of Wisdom advises. That is, a diet rich in fruits, vegetables, beans, grains, and other forms of plants. As evidence of this, studies have shown that a "Daniel diet" of pulse (plant foods) can yield incredible, clinically-significant improvements in all aspects of health.[49] These health benefits are blessings that we can't live without in today's world rife with chronic disease. The Lord also encourages us to eat these foods while they are "in season."[50] Modern data confirm the benefit of following this counsel as well, showing that the nutrient profiles of in-season foods are far greater than when out of season.[51]

---

[48] Huaidong Du et al., "Fresh fruit consumption and all-cause and cause-specific mortality: findings from the China Kadoorie Biobank." *International journal of epidemiology,* vol. 46, no. 5, 2017, pp. 1444-55.

[49] Richard J Bloomer et al., "Effect of a 21 day Daniel Fast on metabolic and cardiovascular disease risk factors in men and women." *Lipids in health and disease,* vol. 9, no. 94, 3 September 2010.

[50] Doctrine and Covenants 89:11.

[51] J.H. Everitt and C.L. Gonzalez, "Seasonal Nutrient Content in Food Plants of White-tailed Deer on the South Texas Plains," *Journal of Range Management,* vol. 4, no. 6, November 1981.

We ought to remember that the Lord also directs us to use these with "prudence and thanksgiving."[52] Therefore, we should use judgment when partaking of these foods to ensure that they are used for improved health and not to our detriment. As President Joseph Fielding Smith reminds us, "Any perfect food that is good for the body, can be harmful by over-indulgence."[53] So let us remember that there can be too much of a good thing, and we should strive to not overindulge in *any* kind of food, even the most wholesome.

Man's wisdom is not greater than God's and we ought to rely wholly upon His wisdom. As we obey these principles, we *will* be rewarded. There can be untold miracles of healing as we obey the Lord's prescribed way. When we use the foods that He has ordained, we can grow in both spirit and strength of body. No matter where you currently are on your journey, finding ways to add in more of these prescribed foods can be a great blessing.

Healing Disease with Diet

When talking about the Word of Wisdom, we often miss the "dos." These important foods ordained for our constitution, nature, and use can have miraculous healing powers. For instance, broccoli has been shown to kill colon cancer cells on site.[54] Berries can turn off inflammation genes within a few weeks of consistent consumption.[55] Dark leafy greens are the most nutrient-dense foods on the planet, and play a critical role

---

[52] Doctrine and Covenants 89:11

[53] Joseph Fielding Smith, *Answers to Gospel Questions*, (Salt Lake City, UT: Deseret Book Company, 1957), p 201.

[54] L Gamet-Payrastre et al., "Sulforaphane, a naturally occurring isothiocyanate, induces cell cycle arrest and apoptosis in HT29 human colon cancer cells." *Cancer research*, vol. 60, no. 5, 2000, pp. 1426-33.

[55] Anand R Nair et al., "Blueberry supplementation attenuates oxidative stress within monocytes and modulates immune cell levels in adults with metabolic syndrome: a randomized, double-blind, placebo-controlled trial." *Food & function*, vol. 8, no. 11, 2017, pp. 4118-28.

in preventing and reversing heart disease.[56] Soy has been shown to protect against prostate and breast cancer and can even "turn off" the BRCA gene.[57] The list goes on and on.

As I (Cassidy) began my journey to health, I used food exclusively to reverse my health woes. I had yet to learn about herbs (which we'll talk about next), and I didn't use any supplements or medications. I simply used God's food to heal my body. Just as important as what I didn't put into my body–specifically meat, processed foods and other animal products–were what I did put in: fruits, vegetables, grains, seeds, nuts, beans, and legumes. Each of these foods has healing properties and played a role in reversing my disease. Since that time I have worked with people all over the world to help reverse their health conditions. Using only food, I have helped many people reverse some of the most common lifestyle diseases around.

For example, I work with many clients who suffer from severe IBD and IBS, such as Crohn's Disease and Colitis. For these specific conditions, foods like potatoes, brown rice, and steamed vegetables can help promote healing the most. One client had been diagnosed with severe Crohn's disease and Colon cancer. With initial reluctance, she started the dietary recommendations and began her diet of potatoes, rice, and a few other approved items. Within weeks she said that her bloating had subsided, all abdominal pain disappeared, blood in the stool was gone for the first time since her diagnosis, and she finally had energy to make it throughout the day. She was so elated to have healthy bowel movements without planning her whole life around trips to the bathroom! Her example truly shows how the right kinds of food can heal our bodies. These are the blessings available to us when we make an intentional effort to follow the

---

[56] Danijel Brkić et al., "Nitrate in Leafy Green Vegetables and Estimated Intake." *African journal of traditional, complementary, and alternative medicines*, vol. 14, vol. 3, 2017, pp. 31-41.
[57] Rémy Bosviel et al., "Can soy phytoestrogens decrease DNA methylation in BRCA1 and BRCA2 oncosuppressor genes in breast cancer?," *Omics : a journal of integrative biology*, vol. 16, no. 5, 2012, pp. 235-44.

admonitions about what we *should* put into our bodies rather than only focusing on what we *shouldn't*.

Chapter Seven

The Lord's Pattern of Healing

*"Is any sick among you? let him call for the
elders of the church; and let them pray over
him, anointing him with oil in the name of
the Lord: And the prayer of faith shall save
the sick, and the Lord shall raise him up . . ."*
James 5:14-15

The Miracle at Hawn's Mill

In the fall of 1838, tensions between Missouri residents and
the influx of Saints ran high. On October 27, Missouri Governor
Liliburn Boggs issued his infamous extermination order of the
"Mormons," stating: "The Mormons must be treated as enemies
and must be exterminated or driven from the state, if necessary
for the public good. Their outrages are beyond all description."[1]
The very next day a mob of over 200 armed men rode into a
settlement known as Hawn's Mill and massacred the Saints
living there. This band of ruffians with painted faces paid no
attention to the pleas of peace and mercy from the residents.
Many men and boys crowded inside the blacksmith shop to take
up a defense against the persecutors. However, the mob
overpowered these Saints and fired upon the building from all
sides until there was no return fire. They then went into the shop
and shot each person they thought might not be dead. In all,
nearly 20 people were murdered in the Hawn's Mill incident.[2]

---

[1] Joseph Smith, *History of the Church*, vol. 3, p. 175.
[2] Ibid, p. 176.

Despite this awful scene of bloodshed, the Lord showed forth His wisdom and power in a miracle of healing.

Willard Smith, whose father and younger brother Sardis lay among the dead, recorded finding another of his brothers, Alma, unconscious but alive among a pile of bodies. When Williard found their mother, Amanda, she placed Alma on a makeshift bed and assessed the damage. As she cut his trousers, she found that the "entire ball and socket of [his] left hip had been shot away leaving the bones about three or four inches apart."[3] When Alma regained consciousness, Amanda informed him of the situation and asked him if he had faith that the Lord could make him a new hip. Alma replied that if she believed the Lord could do it, then he would believe it, too. Mother Amanda then gathered what remained of her family around her wounded Alma and prayed for guidance, dedicating him to the Lord that he would be "restored and made well and strong."[4]

Feeling helpless and afraid of the continued threat of mob violence, Amanda prayed earnestly to know what to do. As her son Willard recorded, her prayers were answered, and she knew exactly what to do by way of inspiration. Taking some ash from the fireplace, she first made a "mild lye solution with which she bathed [Alma's] gaping wound until it was as white as the breast of a chicken, with all the mangled flesh and bone gone."[5] She was then directed to take roots of the slippery elm tree to make a poultice to apply on the wound. Alma lay still in bed for five weeks, and then one day while Amanda was away getting water, she suddenly heard the children screaming from inside the house. As she rushed through the door, she was astonished to see all of her children running around the house with Alma leading the pack. By his faith and the faith of his mother, little

---

[3] Alexander L. Baugh, "A Rare Account of the Haun's Mill Massacre: The Reminiscence of Willard Gilbert Smith," *Mormon Historical Studies*, vol. 8, nos. 1–2, Spring-Fall 2007, p. 167.
[4] Ibid.
[5] Ibid.

Alma was completely healed! Willard recorded that Alma would never experience any pain or discomfort and would even fulfill a mission where he would do a great amount of walking.[6]

What many do not realize about this story is that the method of treatment Amanda Smith pursued to help heal her young son is the exact pattern the Lord prescribes in the Doctrine and Covenants and is directly connected to the Word of Wisdom.

God's Instruction for Healing

In what is considered the "Law of the Church,"[7] the Lord provides a three-step pattern for treating illness and for healing. This pattern is so simple and takes up so few verses that it is very easy to overlook:

> "And whosoever among you are sick, and have not **faith** to be healed, but believe, shall be nourished with all tenderness, with **herbs** and **mild food**, and that not by the hand of an enemy.
>
> And the elders of the church, two or more, shall be called, and shall pray for and lay their hands upon them in my name; and if they die they shall die unto me, and if they live they shall live unto me."[8]

Upon first reading, the pattern may not be so obvious. But on closer inspection, we can begin to see it, as it takes a little work to put it together. The pattern looks like this:

Step 1: Have faith to be healed through prayer and priesthood blessings.

Step 2: Use herbs.

Step 3: Use mild food.

---

[6] Ibid, p. 168.
[7] Doctrine and Covenants 42.
[8] Doctrine and Covenants 42:43-44, emphasis added.

The Prophet Joseph Smith was known to preach these principles often. One instance from his journal reads:

"I preached to a large congregation at the stand, on the science and practice of medicine, desiring to persuade the Saints to trust in God when sick, and not in an arm of flesh, and **live by faith and not by medicine, or poison**; and when they were sick, and had **called for the Elders to pray for them**, and they were not healed, to **use herbs and mild food**."[9]

It is clear from these verses, Joseph's teachings, and the story of Alma Smith, that the Lord intended for His children to rely upon Him when it comes to sickness and injury. Indeed, the Lord has indicated that the first step to wellness ought to be our faith in Him and His power. The next step is to use the plants that God created and ordained for the specific purpose of healing. The last step is to use food that will help soothe the body and reduce inflammation. Despite this simple plan laid out by the Lord, how many of us first turn to prayer, a blessing, or plants when we feel a cold coming on? On the contrary, most of us turn to Ibuprofen, Nyquil, or other, as one might say, 'pharmakeia.' Because our use of these things has replaced what God has counseled, could they be one of the false gods that we are warned about in the scriptures?[10] One of Satan's greatest ways to deceive us is through counterfeit and imitation of God's ways. In this case, it takes the place of God and His healing power. But unlike God's healing, man's creations for healing often come with a list of terms and conditions as well as side effects sometimes equally or even more detrimental than the ailment itself. In this chapter, we will limit our discussion to the first two steps, as the last step of using mild food is largely outlined in the previous chapter.

---

[9] Joseph Smith, *History of the Church*, vol. 4, p. 414, emphasis added.
[10] Exodus 20:3.

"If You Have Faith You Shall Be Healed"

To expound more on the role of faith in our healing, verse 48 of Section 42 promises that "if you have faith you shall be healed," unless it is your appointed time for death.[11] In other words, there is not a single disease that exists on this planet that God cannot heal if only we will have faith enough to make it so. Is this not part of the work that Christ did while in mortality and that His apostles carried on? Surely, we do not need the Savior to be physically present to access His divine power of healing. When a certain Roman centurion's servant fell ill and was near death, the centurion sent for the help of Jesus.[12] But when Jesus approached, the centurion asked his friends to tell Jesus not to enter into his house because he felt he was not worthy. Instead, he asked that Jesus simply "say in a word, and my servant shall be healed."[13] The Lord was so astonished at the faith of this Gentile that he turned to his disciples and followers and said, "I have not found so great faith, no, not in Israel."[14] When the friends of the centurion returned, the servant had been completely healed.

Israel was the Lord's chosen people, and yet it was a Gentile who displayed the greatest amount of faith. It should have been the other way around; it should have been the covenant people exemplifying great faith to the world. This example should help us understand that healing by God's power is not necessarily predicated upon any requirement of physical proximity–only upon faith and the Lord's will.

Scenarios like this are seen over and over throughout the New Testament. The Lord healed Peter's mother-in-law from a deadly fever.[15] He healed the woman with the issue of blood, a disease that had plagued her 12 years, and as the scriptures say,

---

[11] Doctrine and Covenants 42:48.
[12] Luke 7:2-4.
[13] Luke 7:7.
[14] Luke 7:9.
[15] Mark 1:31.

had been made worse by physicians despite giving them all of her money.[16] The Savior raised Jairus's daughter[17] and Lazurus[18] from the dead when it appeared that all hope was lost. He healed the leper immediately.[19] In the New Testament we read that he healed "many that were sick of divers diseases,"[20] and that he "healed *every* sickness and *every* disease among the people."[21]

If Christ can heal all kinds of sickness and raise people from the dead, is there any of our diseases that He can't fix? Jesus told his disciples that they would do greater works than He did if they would believe in Him.[22] Indeed, if it is according to God's will, there is no disease, no pandemic, no ailment, no cancer, no autoimmune disease, no birth defect, that is more powerful than the faith of the righteous.

Why God Ceases to Work Miracles

In our day, many will scoff at this assertion, even among the Latter-day Saints. Instead, they believe in a god who has ceased to do miracles of healing. In the Book of Mormon, Moroni writes about this subject as he finishes the record of his father. In this powerful account, Moroni speaks to all those that "have imagined up unto [themselves] a god who can do no miracles,"[23] and recounts many miracles such as the creation of heaven and the earth, the creation of man, and many miracles wrought by Jesus and His apostles.[24] He then asks this question: "And if there were miracles wrought then, why has God ceased to be a God of miracles and yet be an unchangeable Being?"[25] In other words, if God healed man through faith and the power of the

---

[16] Mark 5:25-29.
[17] Mark 5: 4.
[18] John 11: 43-44.
[19] Matthew 8:2-3.
[20] Mark 1:34.
[21] Matthew 9:35, emphasis added.
[22] John 14:12.
[23] Mormon 9:15.
[24] Mormon 9:17-18.
[25] Mormon 9:19.

priesthood, why is that not the case now? Moroni gives the answer:

". . . behold, I say unto you he changeth not; if so he would cease to be God; and he ceaseth not to be God, and is a God of miracles. And the reason why he ceaseth to do miracles among the children of men is **because that they dwindle in unbelief, and depart from the right way, and know not the God in whom they should trust.**"[26]

According to Moroni, there are three reasons why God would cease to do miracles, and for our discussion, heal. These reasons are unbelief, departing from the right way, and not knowing God. Unbelief would appear to be the most understood reason for a lack of miracles, which is similar to not having a correct knowledge of God, but the latter can easily be remedied by study and faith. But what about departing from the right way? Certainly, this is likely caused by unbelief. But could departing from the right way mean that we stray from the Lord's revealed patterns and commandments? If we stray from the things God has commanded in scripture, including healing, are we to believe that we will obtain a miracle? On the other hand, if we follow the counsel the Lord has provided with the faith of the centurion, we will receive the miracle, given it is not our time to leave mortality.

Herbs as Medicine in the Scriptures

After we put forward our faith in the Lord and His power, the next step to healing is to use herbs. As we discussed in the last chapter, the word "herbs" can refer to all kinds of plants. However, in Doctrine and Covenants 42, it's clear that the Lord isn't talking about apples or pears. Instead, He refers to the kinds of herbs that can be used as seasonings and for healing purposes. We confess that for much of our lives, we knew little

---

[26] Mormon 9:19-20, emphasis added.

about herbs and their role in health, thinking they were fringe methods only used by witch doctors and snake oil salesmen. However, we were surprised to learn of their use throughout history and the scriptures. Surely, an often undiscussed part of the Word of Wisdom is the use of and need for herbs. Throughout scripture, the Lord repeatedly advises the use of these kinds of herbs. On one occasion He said:

> "Yea, and the herb . . . [is] made for the benefit and the use of man, both to please the eye and to gladden the heart; Yea, for food and for raiment, for taste and for smell, **to strengthen the body and to enliven the soul**. And it pleaseth God that he hath given all these things unto man."[27]

Just as we learn in the Word of Wisdom, these verses state that herbs are made for our use as food and a multitude of other purposes. The Word of Wisdom states that herbs are for our constitution and use, which definitions would naturally include healing. Indeed, these plants entice our senses and give strength to not only our physical bodies but to our spirits as well.

Interestingly enough, advocacy for the use of herbs as medicine can be found throughout each of the standard works. The Psalmist advises the use of Hyssop for purging illness.[28] Ezekiel says that leaves are for medicine.[29] King Nebuchadnezzar recovered from his insanity by eating the herbs of the field.[30] Paul counseled the Romans to eat herbs when they were weak.[31] In the Book of Mormon, we learn that many of the people did not die of illness, "because of the excellent qualities of **the many plants and roots** which God had prepared **to remove the cause of diseases**, to which men were subject by the

---

[27] Doctrine and Covenants 59:17-20, emphasis added.
[28] Psalm 51:7.
[29] Ezekiel 47:12.
[30] Daniel 4:33-34.
[31] Romans 14:2.

nature of the climate."[32] Furthermore, we counted over 42 references in the Bible about herbal remedies. Remedies such as aloe,[33] cinnamon,[34] coriander,[35] cumin,[36] garlic,[37] mint,[38] juniper,[39] and rose[40] are just a few of the ones mentioned throughout the Bible. It is clear that the scriptures are replete with examples of various forms of herbs being used for health and healing beginning with Adam and Eve, being used in Christ's day, and even being mentioned in the Doctrine and Covenants.

Within the Word of Wisdom itself, we are told that barley is a useful herb in mild drinks. Unsurprisingly, barley has many health benefits and has been used for thousands of years across nearly every culture and civilization as an elixir and remedy. Simple barley water has been shown as a powerful detoxifier and digestive aid.[41]

The Prophet and Herbs

The Prophet Joseph Smith may have been one of the biggest advocates of herbal medicine. Speaking of one of the most famous herbalist in America at the time, Samuel Thomson, he allegedly said that Thomson was "as much inspired to bring forth his principle of practice according to the dignity and importance of it as I was to introduce the Gospel."[42] This kind of reverence for the practice of herbal medicine is indicative of its importance not only to the Saints but to the Lord. As we have

---

[32] Alma 46:40, emphasis added.
[33] Numbers 24:6.
[34] Exodus, 30:23, Revelations 18:13.
[35] Numbers 11:7.
[36] Isaiah 28:25.
[37] Numbers 11:5.
[38] Matthew 23:23, Luke 11:42.
[39] 1 Kings 19:4-5.
[40] Luke 11:42.
[41] Plavaneeta Borah, "5 Amazing Barley Water Benefits: Drink Up This Elixir to Good Health," NDTV Food, 30 August 2018.
[42] J. Cecil Alter, "Journal of Priddy Meeks," *Utah Historical Quarterly,* Utah State Historical Society, 1942, vol. 10, p. 199.

already noted, Joseph recorded multiple instances in his journal when he preached about, used, and administered herbs to the Saints. One particular entry Joseph recorded reads:

> "I awoke this morning in good health, but was soon suddenly seized with a great dryness of the mouth and throat; sickness of the stomach, and vomited freely; my wife waited on me assisted by my Scribe Dr. Willard Richards and his brother Levi, who administered to me herbs and mild drinks . . . by evening [I] was considerably revived."[43]

This makes sense considering that, Joseph called Levi and Willard Richards, prominent herbalists in the area, as herbal doctors in Nauvoo. Joseph remarked that Levi Richards was one of the greatest doctors he had ever known.[44] One account suggests that Joseph did not allow any mainstream doctors of the day to even practice in Nauvoo.[45] Even Brigham Young continued to preach the pattern of healing laid out by the Lord and the Prophet. On one occasion he said:

> "If you are sick, **live by faith** and let surgeon's medicine alone. If you want to live, use only such **herbs and mild food** as are at your disposal. If you give heed to this counsel, you will prosper; but if not, we cannot be responsible for the consequences."[46]

It is clear from scriptures and historical accounts in the early Church that herbs were to be an essential aspect of health and healing. However, it appears that we have largely forgotten this

---

[43] "History, 1838–1856, volume E-1 [1 July 1843–30 April 1844]," p. 1804, The Joseph Smith Papers.

[44] "History, 1838–1856, volume D-1 [1 August 1842–1 July 1843]," p. 1537, The Joseph Smith Papers.

[45] John Heinerman, *Joseph Smith and Herbal Medicine*, (Monrovia, CA: Majority of One Press, 1980), p. 37.

[46] Letter to Captain Jefferson Hunt, Brigham Young office files, 1832-1878 (bulk 1844-1877); General Correspondence, Outgoing, 1843-1876; 1846 August; Church History Library.

counsel over time in favor of the philosophies and wisdom of the world. Indeed, herbs have been used for thousands of years in nearly every single culture to heal all kinds of ailments.[47] It should come as no surprise, then, to learn that nearly every drug on the market was originally derived from an herbal source.[48] Aspirin was derived from Aspirae or Meadowsweet. Morphine was derived from Poppy. Valium was derived from Valerian Root. Cocaine was derived from Coca leaf. Codeine was derived from Wild Cherry Bark. Quinine was derived from Magnolia Bark and Dogwood. Herbs are not new or fringe, they are simply underutilized. Many studies indicate that herbs are an incredible source of healing for every illness imaginable.[49]

Interestingly enough, one of the most famous herbalists in the world also happened to be a member of the Church, Dr. John Christopher. At a young age, Dr. Christopher was diagnosed with serious health problems and was told he would not live past the age of 30. This set him on a quest to learn how to heal his conditions with what God had made rather than what man had made. Over the years, Dr. Christopher has influenced millions (including the authors of this book) to find greater health and healing.

The Power of Herbs

It should be apparent by now that herbs ought to be used with far more frequency than they presently are. Not only has the Lord made clear that herbs are ordained for our use, but modern data confirm their efficacy. Many studies show that in head-to-head trials, herbs *outperform* modern medicine. One

---

[47] Thordur Sturluson, "History of Herbal Medicine," The Herbal Resource, 30 January 2014.

[48] Si-Yuan Pan et al., "New Perspectives on How to Discover Drugs from Herbal Medicines: CAM's Outstanding Contribution to Modern Therapeutics," *Evidence-based complementary and alternative medicine, eCAM*, vol. 2013, 2013, p. 627375.

[49] Lien-Chai Chiang et al., "Antiviral activities of extracts and selected pure constituents of Ocimum basilicum," *Clinical and experimental pharmacology & physiology*, vol. 32, no. 10, 2005, pp. 811-6.

study found that ashwagandha was more effective than hydrocortisone at reducing inflammation.[50] Another study indicated that hops were just as effective for pain management as ibuprofen.[51] Chamomile has been proven to treat ulcers and lower acidity in the stomach more than antacids.[52] Passionflower is found to be equally as effective as oxazepam (Serax) for treating anxiety.[53] The list goes on and on, but the idea remains the same. When it comes to treating a health problem, there is often an herb that can perform the same function as its doctor-prescribed counterpart.

What many are surprised to learn is that many of the plants that we consider "weeds" that grow along the sides of the road and in our yards are highly potent herbs with incredible medicinal value. Those pesky weeds you spend hours picking just may save your life. For instance, plantain leaves (which you likely have in your backyard right now) have anti-inflammatory, analgesic, antibiotic, and immune-stimulating properties.[54] It provides relief for bee stings and insect bites, and it can stop the itching of poison ivy and other allergic reactions.[55] On one occasion while working in our orchard, our son was stung by a

---

[50] Lakshmi-Chandra Mishra et al., "Scientific Basis for the Therapeutic Use of Withania somnifera (Ashwagandha): A Review," *Alternative Medicine Review*, vol. 5, no. 4, pp. 334-46.

[51] M. Lindahl and C. Tagesson, 'Flavonoids as phospholipase A2 inhibitors: importance of their structure for selective inhibition of group II phospholipase A2', Inflammation, vol. 21(3), 1997, pp. 347–56.

[52] M. T. Khayyal, et al., "Mechanisms involved in the gastro-protective effect of STW 5 (Iberogast) and its components against ulcers and rebound acidity," *Phytomedicine : international journal of phytotherapy and phytopharmacology*, vol. 13 Suppl. 5, 2006, pp. 56-66.

[53] S-M Elsas et al., "Passiflora incarnata L. (Passionflower) extracts elicit GABA currents in hippocampal neurons in vitro, and show anxiogenic and anticonvulsant effects in vivo, varying with extraction method." Phytomedicine : international journal of phytotherapy and phytopharmacology vol. 17, no. 12, 2010, pp. 940-9.

[54] P Ravi Tejeshwar Reddy et al., "Antibacterial and anti-inflammatory properties of Plantago ovata Forssk. leaves and seeds against periodontal pathogens: An in vitro study," *Ayu* vol. 39, no. 4, 2018, pp. 226-229.

[55] John R. Christopher, *School of Natural Healing*, (Springville, UT: Christopher Publications, 2005), pp. 52-4.

bee. His hand began to swell up so we had him immediately begin chewing plantain. Cassidy quickly chewed some as well and made a poultice and put it on the sting. Immediately the swelling stopped and the pain subsided.

Dr. John Christopher once said, "the home without Yarrow will have death therein when the plagues come."[56] Perhaps this is because it has been shown to reduce inflammation and boost immunity, in part because it is a powerful astringent.[57] This "weed" will likely look familiar to you, as we notice it often on walks around the neighborhood. Yarrow can also be used on wounds to stop bleeding and dull pain.[58] Furthermore, it is very useful in treating epilepsy because of its anti-seizure effects.[59]

Many are shocked to find that a simple cup of hot water and 1 teaspoon Cayenne can stop a heart attack within 30 seconds![60] On one occasion, a group of doctors put live heart tissue into a sterile beaker filled with distilled water and cayenne pepper. To the amazement of the doctors, the heart tissue had to be trimmed continually every few days because it grew so rapidly. This experiment lasted an astounding 15 years![61] Cayenne is also

---

[56] "Yarrow, Achillea millefolium; (Compositae)," The Complete Writings of Dr. John R. Christopher, The School of Natural Healing, https://online.snh.cc/files/2100/HTML/100hs_yarrow__achillea_millefolium.htm

[57] Renata Dawid-Pać, "Medicinal plants used in treatment of inflammatory skin diseases," Postepy dermatologii i alergologii, vol. 30, no. 3, 2013, pp. 170-7.

[58] Anna B Livdans-Forret et al., "Menorrhagia: a synopsis of management focusing on herbal and nutritional supplements, and chiropractic," The Journal of the Canadian Chiropractic Association, vol. 51, no. 4, 2007, pp. 235-46.

[59] Mahmoud Hosseini et al., "Antioxidant effect of Achillea wilhelmsii extract on pentylenetetrazole (seizure model)-induced oxidative brain damage in Wistar rats." Indian journal of physiology and pharmacology, vol. 57, vol. 4, 2013, pp. 418-24.

[60] "Cayenne, Capsicum annuum; (Solanaceae)," The Complete Writings of Dr. John R. Christopher, The School of Natural Healing, https://online.snh.cc/files/2100/HTML/100hs_cayenne__capsicum_annuum.htm

[61] Ibid.

very beneficial for IBS patients, helping to reduce symptoms significantly.[62]

Comfrey is sometimes called "Knit-bone" or "Boneset" because of it's incredible ability to heal broken bones.[63] Comfrey contains allantoin which encourages epithelial formation that aids in bone healing.[64] Studies have shown that comfrey taken topically speeds up the recovery process of wounds by about half the time compared to common remedies.[65] Pain and inflammation throughout the body is drastically lowered with the use of comfrey. It has even been found to reduce back pain by 95 percent.[66] Despite comfrey being used for thousands of years by civilizations all over the world, however, the FDA banned the sale of comfrey in 2001, citing concerns over "evidence that implicates these substances as carcinogens."[67] The evidence the FDA alludes to appears to come from a study in 1978 where groups of rats were fed comfrey leaves for over a year or more.[68] The rats then developed liver tumors. There have not been any human trials to confirm this judgment, but just like most things, we wouldn't suggest anyone eat comfrey leaves each day for a year or more anyway.

There are so many herbs all around us that can be used for our benefit. It can be overwhelming to learn about all of them

---

[62] M Bortolotti and S Porta, "Effect of red pepper on symptoms of irritable bowel syndrome: preliminary study," *Digestive diseases and sciences,* vol. 56, no. 11, 2011, pp. 3288-95.

[63] Vibha Singh, "Medicinal plants and bone healing," *National journal of maxillofacial surgery,* vol. 8, vol. 1, 2017, pp. 4-11.

[64] Ibid.

[65] Christiane Staigler, "Comfrey: A Clinical Overview," *Phytotherapy Research,* vol. 26, no. 10, 2012, pp. 1441-48.

[66] B M Giannetti et al., "Efficacy and safety of comfrey root extract ointment in the treatment of acute upper or lower back pain: results of a double-blind, randomised, placebo controlled, multicentre trial," *British journal of sports medicine,* vol. 44, no. 9, 2010, pp. 637-41.

[67] Christine J. Lewis, "FDA Advises Dietary Supplement Manufacturers to Remove Comfrey Products From the Market," U.S. Food and Drug Administration, 6 July 2001.

[68] I Hirono et al., "Carcinogenic activity of Symphytum officinale," *Journal of the National Cancer Institute,* vol. 61, no. 3, 1978, pp. 865-9.

and how to use them. Something that you may find useful is to download a plant identification app on your phone and start identifying herbs and plants you come in contact with. You may be shocked just how many herbs you have in your own backyard!

Objection to Herbs and Mild Food

The most common criticism of this view is that God was only giving to the Saints something for their own time because many contemporary apostles have advocated for the use of modern medicine in conjunction with the prayer of faith. Therefore, as some would say, we may disregard the counsel concerning herbs and mild food. However, we would remind the reader of the importance of measuring *every* man's doctrine against the scriptures. As Joseph Fielding Smith said:

> "It makes no difference what is written or what anyone has said, if what has been said is in conflict with what the Lord has revealed, we can set it aside. My words, and the teaching of any other member of the Church, high or low, if they do not square with the revelations, we need not accept them. Let us have this matter clear. **We have accepted the four standard works as the measuring yardsticks, or balances, by which we measure every man's doctrine.**"[69]

Unfortunately for the critics, there is nothing in the standard works that supports this particular critique. However, we do have many scriptures that support the use of herbs. Therefore, it would not be wise to disregard a principle in the scriptures simply because some of the Brethren have expressed a seemingly contradictory opinion. Until revealed otherwise or stated by the unified voice of the Twelve and the First Presidency, it should stand to reason that the word of the Lord in the scriptures remains valid. This argument also doesn't stand scrutiny when

---

[69] Joseph Fielding Smith, *Doctrines of Salvation*, edited by Bruce R. McConkie, vol. 3, (Salt Lake City, UT: Bookcraft, 1956), p. 203.

we consider that, in many instances, herbs outperform traditional medicine at curing common ailments, as previously discussed.

A Personal Experience

As we were in the middle of writing this book, Jordan experienced a most unfortunate event. I (Jordan) was helping people move some tables and chairs for an event, and as I was unloading a table from the back of a trailer, the table slipped and crushed my right big toe. Having broken many other bones in my youth, I knew immediately that this was going to be another. The pain was excruciating, but I didn't want to make a scene over something as small as a toe, so I quietly but slowly limped along with the task. When I arrived home, I took off my shoe and sock to discover a blackening toenail with blood seeping from underneath.

Because I knew the toe was broken, I didn't want to go see a doctor only to have them confirm it and then not do much in the way of treatment (as I had learned from my previous experiences). Cassidy had learned quite a bit over the last few years about the use of herbs for healing, so I wanted to try that route. Unfortunately, she was out of town with our kids and I was home alone, so I called her to inform her of the situation. My parents quickly came over; my dad gave me a blessing; and my mom helped me make an herbal paste with Cassidy's instruction to help bring the swelling down and relieve the pain.

Twenty-four hours went by, and the bleeding continued, although at a much slower pace. When Cassidy arrived home, we went to a chiropractor to see if we could find out specifically where the bone was broken. An ultrasound indicated that there were at least two fractures, one on either side of the toe. By our estimation, the bone under the toenail had probably broken in such a way that it had punctured the skin from the inside, which is what caused the continued bleeding. Many friends and family suggested an X-Ray, in which case the doctors would have certainly recommended surgery. We had followed the Lord's pattern of healing outlined in Doctrine and Covenants 42 so far, but now we were at a crossroads. Should we continue down the path we started and practice the principles we had come to believe? Or should we go the more traditional (and more expensive) route of pain meds, doctors, and surgery?

We carefully considered both options and weighed the implications of each. Taking it to the Lord in prayer, we decided to continue with our plan of herbs and mild food. I will admit that my faith in using herbs to heal a broken bone was weak. But, as Alma says, I had a desire to believe and was willing to give it a shot.[70] We followed a strict treatment of soaking my foot in comfrey tea during the day and then applying a paste of comfrey, wheat germ oil, and honey directly on the injury at night. One of the benefits of this paste is that it seeps into the skin and stimulates the cells to speed up the healing process. Dr. Christopher's Complete Tissue and Bone formula was taken orally several times each day along with herbal calcium tea, which was composed of shavegrass, oat straw, and lobelia. Within a week of this consistent treatment, the pain in my toe subsided and there were signs of healing. Admittedly, however, there were many times where I questioned what I was doing, thinking myself to be crazy. It wasn't until I gave up my doubts and put my trust in the Lord that the healing process started to take off at a rapid pace. Within a few weeks, I was able to put pressure on my toe again and resume walking. To illustrate for the reader what a miracle this was, I went from not even being able to touch the skin of my toe in the slightest without pain to putting full pressure on it and walking in a matter of weeks. The typical recovery time for this type of injury was projected to be two to three months, but we were able to cut the time in half! I firmly believe that because we followed this path, my recovery was not only quicker but more complete as well.

---

[70] Alma 32:27-28.

None of this is to suggest that healing would not have taken place had I followed the more traditional route of painkillers and surgery. Neither should any of this be taken as justification to speak poorly of any skilled and knowledgeable medical professional. As mentioned earlier, I had broken several bones in my youth, all of which had healed via the traditional route. Could I have healed this time by following the wisdom of the world? I believe so. However, Cassidy and I believed this was an opportunity to "live by faith and not by medicine," as the Prophet Joseph Smith taught. As a result, not only did healing occur, but both of us had a significant increase of faith in the Savior and His ways.

With God, All Things Are Possible

It may often seem that the easiest route is to put our faith in doctors and modern medicine to resolve our health woes, but this is not the Lord's way. He has laid out a direct path to getting well and has echoed it in the scriptures and the words of His prophets. He tells us: faith, herbs, and mild food.

When we have enough faith and trust in God, anything is possible! There is no disease or even injury that is too difficult for Christ to heal. Despite what doctors, family members, or others may say, there is nothing too far gone for Christ to heal. Christ may not be here in the flesh, but He has told us that those who believe in Him would do even greater works than He did. The state of health in the world may perhaps be best understood as a reflection of the lack of faith that we have in the Savior.

Some may say, "I wish I had that much faith, but I am not there yet," and that is okay! The Lord loves us and wants to heal us, which is why He prescribes herbs and mild foods alongside our faith and even lack thereof. Herbs in and of themselves contain incredible healing compounds that have been used for thousands of years in nearly every single civilization. Investing time and energy into learning about herbs and how we can practically use them with "prudence" is a worthwhile endeavor.[71] As we do this, we will see incredible changes. Food is just as important because taking herbs won't do us well if we turn around and feed our bodies with that which works against us. Combined faith, herbs, and mild food can cure any ailment that one could encounter while in this mortal probation. If you have doubts as we once did, study it out, take it to the Lord, then experiment upon the word for yourself.

---

[71] Doctrine and Covenants 89:11.

Chapter Eight

The Destroying Angel

*"Prepare ye, prepare ye for that which is to
come, for the Lord is nigh;"*
Doctrine and Covenants 1:12

Ancient Israel and the Destroying Angel

In the book of Exodus, we learn about how God delivered
Israel from the hands of Pharaoh and led them toward the
promised land. The story begins with Moses, who had just
returned from his 40-year journey in the wilderness with a
message for Pharaoh–the phrase we all know so well, "Let my
people go."[1] The Lord had instructed Moses to free the Israelites
from Egyptian bondage. After he, through Aaron, demanded
their release, Pharaoh angrily responded that he would never
free the Hebrew slaves. In response, the Lord instructed Moses
to stretch forth his rod into the water to turn the water to blood.[2]
Still, Pharaoh disbelieved and refused to let the people go.

This scene played out nine times over, and each time a new
plague was released on Egypt. Locusts destroyed the crops,[3]
frogs came in droves,[4] boils infected the people,[5] and even fire
rained down from heaven.[6] Each time, Moses implored Pharaoh

---

[1] Exodus 7:16.
[2] Exodus 7:20.
[3] Exodus 10:14.
[4] Exodus 8:6.
[5] Exodus 9:10.
[6] Exodus 9:23-24.

to release the Israelites and free Egypt from these horrific plagues, but Pharaoh only grew more angry and obstinate. In a final attempt, Moses begged Pharaoh to let the Israelites free, to which Pharaoh hardened his heart and threatened to kill Moses. Moses entreated him, but then prophesied of the final plague that would soon cause untold pain and death. This time, it was not just another plague; this last affliction was the destroying angel.[7]

Moses then gave the Israelites the sign each family would need to be spared: the blood of an unblemished, firstborn lamb.[8] It was to be painted upon the door frames of each of their homes.[9] Each family who did this would be spared their firstborn child; those who did not, had no such promise.[10]

At midnight, the destroying angel arrived.[11] We are told in this account that none were spared but the righteous who had the token of blood above their doorpost. The scriptures say that "there was a great cry in Egypt; for there was not a house where there was not one dead."[12] This event has since been known as the "Passover."

After this scene of sorrow and death, Pharaoh tells the Israelites to leave. Finally, as the Lord had foretold, His people were free. Then the miracle of the parting of the Red Sea occurred, where Moses took the Israelites through on dry ground, just before the waters swept away the pursuing Egyptians. At last, the people were free from the bondage and burdens that they had endured for so long. They were free to worship, gather, and receive the law. After years, they were finally free from the grasps of their oppressors.

---

[7] Exodus 12:23.
[8] Exodus 12:5,13.
[9] Exodus 12:7.
[10] Exodus 12:13.
[11] Exodus 12:29.
[12] Exodus 12:30.

A Pattern in All Things

This story, while both sad and triumphant, is far more than just a nice history lesson. Rather, it could be an *important* and *relevant* history lesson. In the course of our study of the Word of Wisdom, we discovered some interesting passages that lead us to believe that this history will repeat itself at least in some fashion. Central to understanding this is, of course, the Word of Wisdom.

President George Albert Smith perhaps admonished the Saints to figure this out when he said, "Let me plead with you, search the Word of Wisdom prayerfully. **Do not just read it, search it prayerfully.** Discover what our Heavenly Father gave it for."[13] This implies that although the Lord is direct, the meaning is not necessarily spelled out. It requires study, meditation, and prayer. Surely, the Lord gave the Word of Wisdom for our health and for greater capacity to feel the Spirit, as we have already discussed. But what if the Word of Wisdom was also given to save us from the death and destruction in the last days?

In Doctrine and Covenants 52, the Lord tells us, "I will give unto you a pattern in all things.[14] . ." Indeed, the writings of Isaiah are filled with patterns and passages that applied both to the Savior's first coming as well as His second. Patterns are evident throughout prophecy and the standard works. Perhaps the children of Israel and their flight from Egypt represent a pattern for the Lord's modern covenant people.

This case is strengthened even further when we turn to the scriptures and find that the pattern is even more apparent. In our study, we found that many of the ancient plagues released upon Egypt will again be released upon the world in the last days.

---

[13] George Albert Smith, *Conference Report*, April 1949, p. 191, emphasis added.
[14] Doctrine and Covenants 52:14.

Water to Blood[15]

Revelation 16:3-4 – "And the second angel poured out his vial upon the sea; and **it became as the blood of a dead man**: and every living soul died in the sea.

And the third angel poured out his vial upon the rivers and fountains of waters; and **they became blood**."[16]

Frogs[17]

Revelation 16:13 – "And I saw three unclean spirits like **frogs** come out of the mouth of the dragon, and out of the mouth of the beast, and out of the mouth of the false prophet."[18]

Flies[19]

Doctrine and Covenants 29:18 – "Wherefore, I the Lord God will send forth **flies** upon the face of the earth, which shall take hold of the inhabitants thereof, and shall eat their flesh, and shall cause maggots to come in upon them;"[20]

Sores[21]

Revelation 16:2 – "And the first went, and poured out his vial upon the earth; and there fell a noisome and **grievous sore** upon the men which had the mark of the beast, and upon them which worshipped his image."[22]

Hail and Fire[23]

Revelation 8:7 – "The first angel sounded, and there followed **hail and fire** mingled with blood, and they were

---

[15] Exodus 7:20-25.
[16] Revelation 16:3-4, emphasis added.
[17] Exodus 8:5-7.
[18] Revelation 16:13, emphasis added.
[19] Exodus 8:20-24.
[20] Doctrine and Covenants 29:18, emphasis added.
[21] Exodus 9:8-12.
[22] Revelation 16:2, emphasis added.
[23] Exodus 9:22-26.

cast upon the earth: and the third part of trees was burnt up, and all green grass was burnt up."[24]

Locusts[25]
Revelation 9:3 – "And there came out of the smoke **locusts** upon the earth: and unto them was given power, as the scorpions of the earth have power."[26]

Darkness[27]
Revelation 8:12 – "And the fourth angel sounded, and the third part of the sun was smitten, and the third part of the moon, and the third part of the stars; so as the third part of them was darkened, and **the day shone not** for a third part of it, and the night likewise."[28]

Destroying Angel[29]
Doctrine and Covenants 89:21 – "And I, the Lord, give unto them a promise, that the **destroying angel** shall pass by them, as the children of Israel, and not slay them. Amen."[30]

The similarities are indeed striking. However, it is important to note that not all of the plagues mentioned in Exodus can be found in scripture about the last days; nor does the book of Exodus contain *all* of the plagues and signs that will be poured out upon the world in the last days. But, again, perhaps this is a pattern given for our instruction.

The Destroying Angel

If we are to follow this pattern, we would reasonably believe that the destroying angel of the last days will be a final event of many of the plagues and destructions sent down from heaven before modern Israel is led to greater freedom and happiness.

---

[24] Revelation 8:7, emphasis added.
[25] Exodus 10:12-15.
[26] Revelation 9:3, emphasis added.
[27] Exodus 10:21-23.
[28] Revelation 8:12, emphasis added.
[29] Exodus 12:29-30.
[30] Doctrine and covenants 89:21, emphasis added.

With this in mind, perhaps none of the blessings contained in the Word of Wisdom have as far reaching effect as the one stated in verse 21. It bears repeating: "And I, the Lord, give unto them a promise, that the destroying angel shall pass by them, **as the children of Israel,** and not slay them."[31]

When most of us read this, we think that the Lord is speaking symbolically and that the phrase "destroying angel" is a reference to general disease and early death. While this may be true—if we keep the Word of Wisdom we *will* have greater health and will be spared from many diseases and early death—the Lord was speaking literally. There are two obvious reasons for this. First, as we discussed in the first chapter of this book, Joseph Smith recorded that we should take the Word of Wisdom literally; it means what it says. Second, after saying that the destroying angel would pass by, the Lord gives reference to the children of Israel, who had a literal destroying angel pass by them to free them from the oppression of the Egyptians. The Lord specifically points out the pattern!

What is interesting to note about this verse is that the Lord is specifically saying what *He* promises. It's almost as if the promised blessings preceding this one are simply the natural consequences of following the principles. If we follow these principles we will naturally have health and strength. This makes sense considering that Joseph Smith taught that consequences and blessings are tied to God's laws.[32] But with this particular promise, the Lord appears to say that *He* will protect us from the destroying angel; this promise is different than the others.

Modern Prophets Agree

The idea of a literal destroying angel is not only our perspective but the perspective of modern prophets as well. For example, President Harold B. Lee taught about the magnitude of the Word of Wisdom and this verse when he said:

---

[31] Ibid.
[32] Doctrine and Covenants 130:20-21.

"The Lord's word of wisdom counsels the simple diet of fruits, grains and vegetables in season. . . If by faith in this great law, you refrain from the use of food and drink harmful to your bodies, **you will not become a ready prey to scourges that shall sweep the land, as in the days of the people of Moses in Egypt, bringing death to *every* household that has not heeded the commandments of God.**"[33]

Another prophet, namely Ezra Taft Benson, echoed the same thought: "The Lord has **set loose the angels to reap down the earth,** but those who obey the Word of Wisdom along with the other commandments are assured 'that the destroying angel shall pass by them, as the children of Israel, and not slay them.'"[34] Similarly, Elder Brigham Young Jr. taught of a literal destroying angel in connection with the Word of Wisdom. He said:

"How many of us have disregarded [the Word of Wisdom], in every particular? It is to be found on page 240 of the Doctrine and Covenants, and it shadows to me that a time will come in the midst of this people when a **desolating scourge will pass through our ranks,** and the **destroying angel will be in our midst as he was in Egypt** when he slew all the firstborn of the Egyptians. God says 'the destroying angel shall pass by' and shall not harm you if you will observe to do these things."[35]

Some form of a destroying angel or angels will be present in the last days, and the Word of Wisdom is the sign or token needed to be spared just as ancient Israel had their sign. Current

---

[33] Clyde J. Williams, *The Teachings of Harold B. Lee,* (Salt Lake City, UT: Deseret Book Company, 2015), pp. 205-6, emphasis added.
[34] Ezra Taft Benson, "Prepare Ye," General Conference, October 1973, emphasis added.
[35] Brigham Young, Jr. *Journal of Discourses*, vol. 15, p. 193, emphasis added.

President of the Church Russell M. Nelson previously taught this:

> "At the first passover, the destroying angel did pass over houses that were marked with blood on the doorposts. In our day, the faithful keep the Word of Wisdom. **It is one of our signs unto God** that we are His covenant people."[36]

On another occasion he said:

> "[I]n faith, modern Israel is commanded to obey the Word of Wisdom. **It becomes our token of a covenant with the Lord**—a spiritual separator of covenant Israel from the rest of the world.[37] . ."

Just as ancient Israel was given a sign to protect against the destroying angel, modern Israel has also been given a sign. Doctrine and Covenants 89 is the *only place* in Holy Scripture that we are given a promise of protection against this destroying angel. The only other time an offer of protection against this coming plague is given to us in all of the Restored Gospel is in the temple. It ought, then, to be understood by each of us that this is an extremely important matter for us to consider.

Modern Israel's Freedom From Oppression

With ancient Israel, the destroyer paved the way for Moses to lead the children of Israel to the promised land. If we follow the pattern, perhaps the same could be said for modern Israel. The Israelites were held captive by the Egyptians and were not able to worship God as they were commanded. It was not until God sent the destroying angel that Pharaoh softened his heart and let God's people go. In our day, Pharaoh and the kingdom of Egypt

---

[36] Russell M. Nelson, "Addiction or Freedom," General Conference, October 1988.
[37] Russell M. Nelson, "Joy Cometh in the Morning," General Conference, October 1986.

could be a representation of the church of the devil. In the Book of Mormon, Nephi tells us that the church of the devil, the "whore of all the earth," will make war with Christ and His Saints.[38] Similarly, in the book of Revelation, John informs us that this "great whore" is known as "Babylon the Great," the enemy of Christ and His saints.[39] It would logically follow, then, that the destroying angel would be what sets the Saints free from the oppression and trials to come in the last days.

If we turn to Doctrine and Covenants 105:15, this appears to be the case: "Behold, **the destroyer I have sent forth to destroy and lay waste mine enemies. . .**"[40] As we keep reading to the end of the verse, the Lord says something interesting: ". . . and not many years hence they shall not be left to pollute mine heritage, and to blaspheme my name upon **the lands which I have consecrated for the gathering together of my saints.**"[41] The land that the Lord is talking about is the land of Missouri where the New Jerusalem will be built. Section 105 was given to the Prophet Joseph Smith in Zion's Camp when, because of the transgressions of the people, they were to "wait for a little season for the redemption of Zion,"[42] which is yet to transpire. Could the Lord be telling us that in the last days the destroyer will pave the way for His people to return to the land of Zion?

This interpretation of destruction sent forth upon the land (specifically America) preceding the establishment of the New Jerusalem appears to be confirmed by the Savior Himself in the Book of Mormon.[43] Speaking of the Gentiles in the land and those of His Church, the Lord told the Nephites, "I will execute vengeance and fury upon them, even as upon the heathen, such

---

[38] 1 Nephi 14:10-13.
[39] Revelation 17:1-5.
[40] Doctrine and Covenants 105:15, emphasis added.
[41] Ibid, emphasis added.
[42] Doctrine and Covenants 105:9.
[43] 3 Nephi 21:14-25.

as they have not heard."[44] After this great destruction, the Lord promises that those who remain and turn to Him will help establish the New Jerusalem.[45] In Egypt, the children of Israel were able to escape the plagues as they followed the commandments given by Moses. So, too, in the last days can the Saints escape the plagues that shall come upon the land if we give heed to what the Lord commands. As the Lord said in Doctrine and Covenants 97:

> **"The Lord's scourge shall pass over by night and by day**, and the report thereof shall vex all people; yea, it shall not be stayed until the Lord come;
>
> Nevertheless, **Zion shall escape if she observe to do all things whatsoever I have commanded her**.
>
> But if she observe not to do whatsoever I have commanded her, I will visit her according to all her works, with sore affliction, with pestilence, with plague, with sword, with vengeance, with devouring fire."[46]

President J. Reuben Clark echoed these verses in conjunction with the Word of Wisdom when he proclaimed:

> "This does not say and this does not mean, that to keep the Word of Wisdom is to insure us against death, for death is, in the eternal plan, co-equal with birth. This is the eternal decree. But **it does mean that the destroying angel**, he who comes to punish the unrighteous for their sins, as he in olden time afflicted the corrupt Egyptians in their wickedness, **shall pass by the Saints, 'who are walking in obedience to the**

---

[44] 3 Nephi 21:21.
[45] 3 Nephi 21:23-24.
[46] Doctrine and Covenants 97:23,25-26, emphasis added.

commandments,' and who 'remember to keep and do these sayings.'"[47]

After the faithful Israelites avoided the plagues and destruction, they were eventually led to the promised land to build a new society. In our day, it may not take 40 years from the time of the destruction to the time Zion is redeemed by the Lord and His people. When will these things come to pass? We don't know. But the Lord has said that "the angels are crying unto the Lord day and night, who are ready and waiting to be sent forth to reap down the fields."[48] How great the importance, then, for us to live the principles contained in the revelation and do it now! The Word of Wisdom is absolutely about the health of our bodies, but it is also a shield of protection for us in the last days. Through this law of health, we are offered specific protection against the destruction preceding the building up of the New Jerusalem. Indeed, it must be that every aspect of the Word of Wisdom is followed before Zion can rise in all her glory. As stated by the Prophet Joseph Smith: "Men must become harmless, before the brute creation; and when men lose their vicious dispositions and cease to destroy the animal race, the lion and the lamb can dwell together, and the sucking child can play with the serpent in safety."[49]

It is quite likely that the plagues and the destroying angel will bring great destruction and upheaval to our society and our way of life. However, all of the pain and sorrow will be swallowed up in the glory of the New Jerusalem. Surely, it will be "a land of peace, a city of refuge, a place of safety for the saints of the Most High God,"[50] where the Lord has said "the power of heaven [shall] come down among them; and **I also will be in the midst**."[51] With the Savior personally present, this truly will

---

[47] J. Reuben Clark, Jr., *Conference Report*, October 1940, pp. 17-18, emphasis added.
[48] Doctrine and Covenants 86:5.
[49] Joseph Smith, *History of the Church*, vol. 2, p. 71.
[50] Doctrine and Covenants 45:66.
[51] 3 Nephi 21:25, emphasis added.

be Zion! Although we don't know when or how exactly these things will take place, one of the simplest steps each of us can take toward preparing for this wondrous event is to live the Word of Wisdom as best as we understand. As Eliza R. Snow reminded us, Zion is where "we shall meet the Savior face to face. The celestial law must be kept by those who go there. **No one can go who does not keep the word of wisdom.**[52] . . ."

Blood on the Doorpost

The Word of Wisdom is so much more than just a dietary code or law for greater health. It is the blood on our doorpost. It is a token of God's covenant people. It is what will separate those who are destroyed and those who are spared, for the Lord has decreed it. *This* is why the Word of Wisdom is so important. *This* is why we hope that each person can better obey the Word of Wisdom.

Every part of the Word of Wisdom matters. It is not simply avoidance of coffee, tea, tobacco, alcohol, and drugs that will give us protection. It is our use of wholesome foods and our avoidance of meat (except in certain times). It is our focus on grains, use of herbs, and so much more. We can only be blessed according to our level of obedience. While many of us may believe that adherence to the list of don'ts may grant us access to the temple, it very well could be that our adherence to *all* of the Word of Wisdom will determine our protection against the destroying angel. Every aspect of Doctrine and Covenants 89 matters, as it could be the very thing that saves us.

There is no effort too extreme, no study too long, no prayer too fervent in our quest to better obey the Word of Wisdom. The blessings from obedience are immeasurable and can be experienced immediately. The clear conscience, the healthy body, the quick mind, and the companionship of the Spirit can be ours if we will but obey. Perhaps no one has expounded on

---

[52] Eliza R. Snow, *Woman's Exponent*, vol. 19, 1890 June - 1891 June; 1891 May 1, pp. 161-168, Church History Library.

the importance of the Word of Wisdom better and more succinctly than Hyrum Smith when he said:

> "Let these things be adhered to. . . so shall we be blessed of the great Jehovah in time and in eternity: we shall be healthy, strong and vigorous: we shall be enabled to resist disease; and wisdom will crown our councils, and our bodies will become strong and powerful. . . we shall prepare ourselves for the purposes of Jehovah for the kingdom of God for the appearance of Jesus in his glory. . . Zion will be exalted, and become the praise of the whole earth."[53]

---

[53] "The Word of Wisdom," *Times and Seasons*, vol. 3, no. 15, 1 June 1842, p. 801.

Afterword

At the beginning of 2020, I (Cassidy) felt strongly that we needed to pull together some sort of Word of Wisdom conference. I was sitting in sacrament meeting one Sunday and had the strongest impression that we needed to do it as soon as possible. We decided to make it a free event with many different speakers just focusing on practical applications of the Word of Wisdom. We were able to pull it together within a month and had a much larger turnout than we expected. Many different speakers provided remarks about several of the topics discussed in this book. The timing proved to be providential, as the spread of COVID-19 shut down states and economies around the United States just weeks later. Many of the people who attended the conference thanked us for putting it on and inquired about when our book would be available. At the time, the book seemed to be just another one of those "forever projects"–always working on it but never finishing. After so many questions, we decided we had to get serious about it.

As we dove in, we continued to learn more and more about scriptural health and the Word of Wisdom, and as such, our resolve to live the Word of Wisdom increased significantly. As members of the Lord's Church, with His revealed word to guide us, we ought to be the healthiest group of people in the world. Sadly, this is not the case. For those of us who have not yet realized the promised blessings of the Word of Wisdom and the related principles of health, we hope that with some of the information provided in this book, you might seek to know what areas of the Word of Wisdom can be improved upon so that you can obtain those blessings for yourself. No matter where we are on our journey, there is always room for improvement and increased obedience. Perhaps that is why the Lord reminded us within the revelation itself that it is "adapted to the capacity of the weak and weakest of saints."[1] Obedience is attainable by *all* saints, even the very weakest of us, but it does require reliance on Him.

Some may feel that all of this information is empowering and insightful while others may feel discouraged and overwhelmed at such an undertaking. We once felt both of these sentiments as we began our journey. Let us not forget that Christ caused the lame to walk, the blind to see. He revived Peter's mother in law. He healed lepers, and He can heal you. Christ even brought Lazarus back from the dead, so our ailments and challenges can be met when we have faith. As Elder Dallin H. Oaks reminded us:

> "The healing power of the Lord Jesus Christ—whether it removes our burdens or strengthens us to endure and live with them like the Apostle Paul—is available for every affliction in mortality."[2]

The Lord is all-powerful and loves each one of us. He can reach out to you where you are and lift you higher. The Lord has asked that each of His Saints live the Word of Wisdom, and as such, He will offer as much grace and aid as any of us need to accomplish it. As we increase our faith, miracles are sure to follow.

As you conclude this book, we invite you to spend some time writing your thoughts in your journal or on a piece of paper. You might have an increased desire to work with the Lord to kick bad habits and substances. You may feel the need to reduce your meat consumption to times of winter, cold, or famine. Or perhaps you will begin to eat more of the things God has emphasized should be in our diet. Perhaps you are already living these principles but still find yourself addicted to desserts (even the healthy kind) and need to work on being free from addiction.

---

[1] Doctrine and Covenants 89:3.
[2] Dallin H. Oaks, "He Heals the Heavy Laden," General Conference, October 2006.

Maybe you do not use herbs as you think you ought to. Or perhaps you feel that you need to change your motivations for eating this way. Regardless of where you are in your journey, make goals that will help you to draw nearer to our Lord and enable you to receive the promised blessings contained in the Word of Wisdom. Write down how you would like to change as a result of the information in this book. Enlist the help of your Father in Heaven. We are confident that as you strive to be obedient and live the Word of Wisdom with exactness, miracles will occur in your life. Told and untold blessings will flow from heaven. We know that you will receive a greater measure of the Spirit than you ever thought possible.

Appendix

There were a few topics related to the Word of Wisdom that we wanted to include in this book, but we didn't quite feel that they fit into the main body as they are somewhat ancillary. Initially we decided to include these topics in another work, but were persuaded to include them as an appendix instead. The following sections are simply to provide additional and interesting information for your consideration.

What About Dairy and Eggs?

The question about eggs and dairy is one of the most difficult questions to answer when it comes to the Word of Wisdom, but one we receive quite frequently. The short answer is: what *about* milk and eggs? The Word of Wisdom doesn't say anything about them, either. Some people believe that because the revelation is silent on the matter, they should be perfectly fine to eat. Others believe that since there is nothing, we should not indulge. Indeed, it is difficult to make the case that if something is not included in a list of dietary guidelines it is compliant or non-compliant. However, there are no scriptures in the standard works that specifically advise the common use of these animal items. In fact, at very best they are silent on our consumption of them. Though some scriptures make mention of dairy or eggs, they are usually either symbolic or about the poor.[1]

One of the most common phrases used to justify the consumption of milk is "milk and honey," a phrase that typically refers to prosperity and abundance. The scriptures are replete with references to milk and honey in all sorts of contexts. In other instances, the reference to milk is a reference to a mother's

---

[1] Isaiah 7:15 states that the Saviour would eat "butter and honey." Rather than setting forth the Lord's diet, this is more of a commentary on the circumstances from which the Lord would come. This is confirmed by footnote 'a' which reads: "Curd and honey—the only foods available to the poor at times."

milk. In his first epistle, Peter says, "As newborn babes, desire the sincere milk of the word, that ye may grow thereby." This is an obvious reference to mother's milk because, at the time, mothers would have fed their children their milk for several years past infancy.

As we discussed throughout the book, the Word of Wisdom contains three categories of substances: the 'dos,' the 'don'ts,' and the 'sometimes.'   The 'dos' are herbs, grains, and other plants; milk and eggs don't fit there. The 'don'ts' are tobacco, hot drinks, alcohol, and drugs. Milk and eggs don't fit there, either. That leaves us with the 'sometimes.' The 'sometimes' consists of beasts and fowls of the air, which accurately describes milk and eggs. Many people even refer to milk as "liquid meat," and perhaps this is more evidence that it should be treated as such. This puts eggs, milk, cheese, and other animal foods in the same category as meat foods, which means we should only turn to these foods when circumstances necessitate.

If we turn back to Doctrine and Covenants 89, we are told that animals "should not be **used**, only in times of winter, or of cold, or famine."[2] Interestingly, the Lord does not say eaten, He says used. What are other ways aside from the obvious meat they provide that they can be used? Their fur, horns, hoofs, eggs, and milk are all ways that they can be used. The footnote of this verse leads us to another where the Lord says they are to be used, "with judgment, not to excess, **neither by extortion**."[3]

Even if you do not buy into the argument that animal byproducts fit in with the 'sometimes' of the Word of Wisdom, we readily admit that the revelation is silent on the use of these products. However, the Lord clearly outlined in the Word of Wisdom and other revelations what *has* been ordained to be eaten. Milk and eggs are *not* included in any of the prescribed foods. So we must ask ourselves, "Why is the Lord silent on this,

---

[2] Doctrine and Covenants 89:13, emphasis added.
[3] Doctrine and Covenants 59:20, emphasis added.

and what else is He silent on?" The Lord is silent on high fructose corn syrup, MSG, preservatives, chips, candy, and many other products. Does this mean that they are in line with the spirit of the Word of Wisdom—that is, to take care of our mortal frame? Certainly not. Perhaps the Book of Mormon prophet Jacob said it best: "O be wise; what can I say more?"[4]

From a simple nutritional standpoint, there is no question as to whether or not we ought to eat these things. The answer is an increasingly accepted "no." All nutrients or health benefits found in animal byproducts can be found in greater abundance, for cheaper, and without the side effects of animal products in the foods found in the 'dos' of the Word of wisdom. To briefly make mention of some of the research behind this claim, eggs cannot legally advertise using the words 'safe' or 'healthy' or 'nutritious;' this is our first hint that they ought to be avoided.[5] Furthermore, studies indicate that eating eggs can be equally as detrimental to your blood vessels as smoking.[6] This in part comes because a single egg has 187 mg of cholesterol.[7] Other studies found that people who eat an egg a day have up to double the risk of developing Type 2 diabetes.[8] And eating five or more eggs a week has been associated with an increased risk of breast, prostate, colon, and ovarian cancers.[9]

---

[4] Jacob 6:12.
[5] Michael Greger, "Who Says Eggs Aren't Healthy or Safe?," *NutritionFacts.org*, vol. 14, 17 February 2014.
[6] J David Spence et al., "Egg yolk consumption and carotid plaque," *Atherosclerosis*, vol. 224, no. 2, 2012, pp. 469-73.
[7] Luc Djoussé and J Michael Gaziano, "Egg consumption in relation to cardiovascular disease and mortality: the Physicians' Health Study," *The American journal of clinical nutrition*, vol. 87, no. 4, 2008, pp. 964-9.
[8] Lina Radzevičienė and Rytas Ostrauskas, "Egg consumption and the risk of type 2 diabetes mellitus: a case-control study," *Public health nutrition*, vol. 15, no. 8, 2012, pp. 1437-41.
[9] Sandi Pirozzo et al., "Ovarian Cancer, Cholesterol, and Eggs," *Cancer Epidemiol Biomarkers Prev*, vol. 11, no. 10, October 2002, pp. 1112-4.

Milk is extremely high in fat (the bad kind)[10] and is directly linked to prostate, breast, and ovarian cancers.[11] Even the most free-range, homegrown cow with no antibiotic use produces milk that is naturally extremely high in bovine hormones, which are directly linked with hormone disruption in humans leading to infertility, PMS, PCOS, and more. Contrary to popular belief, milk also depletes Vitamin C and calcium from bone stores, causing bone fractures.[12] And, most interesting, the groundbreaking "China Study" (one of the largest nutritional studies ever performed) found that you can turn off cancer cells simply by eliminating dairy.[13] Moreover, this study found that cancer cells were reignited when dairy was reintroduced. If this information is not enough, other studies have also shown that over 65 percent of the global population is lactose intolerant.[14] If the Lord intended us to have dairy products, why would so many of his children be allergic to it?

Ultimately, there are substantive arguments to be made on both sides. For example, most of the prophets and apostles ate eggs and dairy throughout their lives. Does this mean they didn't live the Word of Wisdom the "right way"? Of course not. You must therefore use your judgement and the spirit of revelation to decide what to do.

I (Cassidy) experienced the blessings of stopping my consumption of dairy and eggs. On three various occasions throughout my life, I stopped consuming meat for different

---

[10] Tara Martine, "How Is Milk Fat Calculated?," TheNest.com, XO Group Inc.

[11] Dagfinn Aune et al., "Dairy products, calcium, and prostate cancer risk: a systematic review and meta-analysis of cohort studies." *The American journal of clinical nutrition,* vol. 101, no. 1, 2015, pp 87-117. See also Wei Lu et al., "Dairy products intake and cancer mortality risk: a meta-analysis of 11 population-based cohort studies." Nutrition journal, vol. 15, no. 1, 2016, p. 91.

[12] Heike A Bischoff-Ferrari et al., "Milk intake and risk of hip fracture in men and women: a meta-analysis of prospective cohort studies," *Journal of bone and mineral research: the official journal of the American Society for Bone and Mineral Research,* vol. 26, no. 4, 2011, pp. 833-9.

[13] See *The China Study* by T. Colin Campbell and Thomas Campbell.

[14] "Lactose intolerance," Genetics Home Reference, National Institutes of Health, May 2010.

reasons. Though I stopped eating meat, I still ate moderate amounts of eggs and large amounts of dairy. Each time I stopped eating meat, I noticed improved health but my challenges never went away completely. I was still unable to fully claim the promised blessings of health and strength in the Word of Wisdom. Feeling discouraged, I added meat back into my diet each time. I worked hard to ensure I had the cleanest products. I bought all grass-fed, organic, free-range products and always bought raw milk and cheese from a variety of animals.

As Jordan and I learned new things about the Word of Wisdom that we had never considered, we felt that we needed to move to more of a "Daniel diet," that is, to leave aside the meat, eggs, and dairy in favor of the "pulse" or plant foods, unless we found ourselves in dire circumstances. It wasn't until we made this change that the windows of heaven were opened to us and we experienced greater health than we thought was possible; it was like we began to get younger, not older, and our countenances surely showed it. Interestingly enough, one study has shown that a Daniel diet of pulse and water can have incredible, clinically significant improvements in health.[15]

We are not here to tell you how to act regarding dairy and eggs, only to present information and our own experience that you may not have previously considered. But if you are following each of the admonitions in the Word of Wisdom and still do not have the blessings you desire, perhaps this is a perfect opportunity to test out the Daniel diet. Experiment upon the word to see if it is good. By your own experience, you'll be able to know whether this is something you should follow or not. Give it two weeks, and see how you feel. There is certainly nothing to lose, but much to be gained.

---

[15] RJ Bloomer et al., "Effect of a 21 day Daniel Fast on metabolic and cardiovascular disease risk factors in men and women," *Lipids Health Dis.*, vol. 9, September 2010, p. 94.

Christ Drank Wine and Ate Meat

The four gospels of the KJV New Testament give us a brief look at Christ's life. Though these accounts are incredibly important and ought to be studied with great care, they are just a small fragment of the historic and spiritual writings that exist about the life of Jesus of Nazareth. Many additional gospels, historical accounts, alternate translations, and apocryphal books often provide important context and information but did not make it into the KJV. Many members are scared of these books, as their veracity and origins are sometimes questionable. However, it is interesting to note that Joseph Smith often referred to and used other translations of the Bible in his personal studies. One version he would have used contained the apocrypha. Referring to the apocrypha, Doctrine and Covenants Section 91 assures us that many of the things therein are true and it is mostly translated correctly.[16] The Lord goes on to say that we ought to read these things by the Spirit, and the Holy Ghost will manifest to us what of it is true.[17] With this approach in mind, it is exciting for many members to learn that there is a great deal written in other texts about the teachings and personal diet of Jesus Christ. What we offer in this section is a different look at what we find in the English King James Version of the Bible. We do not claim to have discovered any hidden or new doctrines, simply interesting information to consider.

The first major issue with the idea that Jesus drank intoxicating wine is that many of these assertions are from anti-Christians that discuss the use of wine during the time of Christ. So a complete and accurate picture of wine usage is unlikely. That being said, there are some clues in ancient historical texts that help us to understand the situation a little bit better.

As already discussed in chapter 4, it is very clear from many passages in the Bible that intoxicating wine is condemned.[18] One

---

[16] Doctrine and Covenants 91:1.
[17] Doctrine and Covenants 91:4-5.
[18] Ephesians 5:18.

passage indicates that wine was associated with woe, sorrow, contentions, babbling, and redness of eyes.[19] Some historical records indicate that the Jews took great care to store the wine properly so that it did not turn bad but also so that it would not ferment and become alcoholic. It should be remembered that alcoholic wine is not naturally occurring. It is an arduous process that includes the correct amount of water, sugar, time and temperature. So, simply putting wine in a barrel until the next season would not suffice in making it an alcoholic beverage. If this alcoholic form of wine was condemned throughout scripture, we can logically infer that it would not be in Christ's character to defile His body with such things. Some of the quotations below may provide more insight.

As members of the Church, we use a version of the Bible that came from a Greek manuscript. However, the Syriac-Aramaic manuscript is regarded as being more correct by some historians, since it was written in the language that Christ and His disciples would have spoken. In this version of Luke 21, the Lord teaches His disciples:

> "Be on guard, so that your hearts do not become heavy with the **eating of flesh** and with the **intoxication of wine** and with the anxiety of the world, and that day come upon you suddenly; for as a snare it will come upon all who dwell upon the surface of the earth."[20]

Here we see that Jesus specifically counseled against intoxicating drink as well as the eating of meat. Some may ask, how does this square with the portrayals in the New Testament of Christ eating fish? First, it is interesting to note that in the original story of Christ feeding the five thousand, He is said to have fed the crowd with both bread and fish.[21] However, each

---

[19] Proverbs 23:29-31.
[20] Luke 21:34, Evangelion Da-Mepharreshe — Old Syriac-Aramaic Manuscript of the New Testament Gospels, emphasis added.
[21] Matthew 14:13-21.

time Christ retrospectively discusses the event, He makes no mention of fish, only referring to the bread.[22] It would seem that fish was later added to the original story considering the fact that early church writers such as Irenaeus, Eusebius, and Arnobius all wrote of the miracle of feeding the 5000, but made no mention of fish.[23]

Various other works, such as the Hebrew gospels, also portrayed Jesus as not eating any animals–including fish. Other texts from groups such as the Essenes, Nazarenes, and Ebionites all suggest that Christ ate a meat-free diet, some going as far as to advocate that he didn't partake of any animal substances. For some historical background on these groups of people which may be largely unfamiliar to Latter-day Saints, we turn to Dr. James Tabor:

> "Josephus reports four main sects or schools of Judaism: Pharisees, Sadducees, Essenes, and Zealots. The earliest followers of Jesus were known as Nazarenes, and perhaps later, Ebionites, and form an important part of the picture of Palestinian Jewish groups in late 2nd Temple times.
>
> The Ebionite/Nazarene movement was made up of mostly Jewish/Israelite followers of John the Baptizer and later Jesus, who were concentrated in Palestine and surrounding regions and led by 'James the Just' (the oldest brother of Jesus) . . . The term Ebionite (from Hebrew 'Evyonim) means 'Poor Ones' and was taken from the teachings of Jesus: 'Blessed are you Poor Ones, for yours is the Kingdom of God'. . ."[24]

---

[22] Matthew 16:9; see also Mark 8:16-21.
[23] James Bean, "Evidence That Jesus and The Original Aramaic Christians Were Vegetarians," *Inner Tapestry Journal*, 1 January 2018.
[24] James Tabor, "The Jewish Roman World of Jesus," UNC Charlotte, https://pages.uncc.edu/james-tabor/ancient-judaism/nazarenes-and-ebionites/.

Dr. Tabor also explains that Nazarene was probably the first term used for the followers of Christ as mentioned in the Bible.[25] In relation to the use of animal flesh, Jesus is purported to have said in the Gospel of the Nazarenes:

". . .knowest thou not that God in the beginning gave to man the fruits of the earth for food, and did not make him lower than the ox, or the horse, or the sheep, that he should kill and eat the flesh and blood of his fellow creatures."[26]

On another occasion, He taught:

"Wherefore I say unto all who desire to be my disciples, keep your hands from bloodshed and let no flesh meat enter your mouths, for God is just and bountiful, who ordaineth that man shall live by the fruits and seeds of the earth alone."[27]

These ancient texts give us an interesting perspective that our New Testament does not. Even more intriguing, however, are the historical accounts from the early Christian church about the disciples and their followers. There is overwhelming evidence from a variety of sources that the early Apostles did not partake of meat or wine. Many of these accounts originate from early church historian Eusebius. Eusebius, whom one prominent scholar has called the "first great Christian ecclesiastical historian," wrote a ten volume comprehensive history of the early Church.[28] In one of his works, Eusebius writes that the disciples "embraced and persevered in a strenuous and a laborious life, with fasting and abstinence from wine and

---

[25] Ibid, see also Acts 24:5.
[26] The Gospel of the Holy Twelve 28:2, translated by G.J.R. Ouseley, November 2009.
[27] Ibid, 38:4.
[28] W. Cleon Skousen, "The Old Testament Speaks Today," *Ensign*, December 1972.

meat."[29] In his comprehensive history, Eusebius records that this "mode of life . . . has been preserved to the present time by us alone."[30]

In the New Testament we learn that John the Baptist ate locusts. However, a closer look shows that he was a Nazarite, who believed in living an austere and humble lifestyle. The carob bean, also known at the Locust bean, was commonly regarded as one of the most readily available foods eaten by this priestly class. Therefore, it can be reasonably inferred that John likely ate locust *plant* seed from the carob tree, not actual locusts.[31] In fact, according to church historian Hegesippus, John "never ate meat."[32]   But John was not the only one that we likely have incorrect information about.

Other texts indicate that others of the apostles abstained from both meat and wine as well. Peter reportedly said, "I live on olives and bread, and rarely [vegetables]."[33] On another occasion he taught that "The unnatural eating of flesh meats is as polluting as the heathen worship of devils, with its sacrifices and its impure feasts, through participation in it a man becomes a fellow eater with devils."[34] We are told in Acts of Thomas that Thomas abstained from the eating of meat and drinking of wine.[35] Matthew ate only "seeds, and nuts, hard-shelled fruits, and vegetables, without flesh." [36]And most interesting is James, the brother of Jesus. According to Eusebius, James "was holy from his mother's womb; and he drank no wine nor strong

---

[29] Eusebius, *Demonstratio Evangelica* or *Proof of the Gospels*, vol. 3, chapter 5, translated by W.J. Ferrar, 1920.

[30] Eusebius, *Ecclesiastical History*, vol. 2, 17:22, translated by Arthur McGiffert.

[31] Bart D. Ehrman, Lost Christianities: The Battles for Scripture and the Faiths We Never Knew, pp. 102, 103.

[32] Eusebius, Church History Book II, 2:3.

[33] Clementine Homilies 12:6; see also Recognitions 7:6.

[34] Steven Rosen, *Food for the Spirit: Vegetarianism and the World Religions*, (New York: Bala Books 1987), p. 19.

[35] *The Apocryphal New Testament*, Acts of Thomas, verse 20, Translation by M. R. James, (Oxford: Clarendon Press, 1924).

[36] Clement of Alexandria, *Christ the Educator*, (The Fathers of the Church Volume 23), pp. 107-8.

drink, nor did he eat flesh...”[37] This assertion was repeated by St. Augustine who said that James “lived upon seeds and vegetables, never tasting flesh or wine.”[38] Here we learn that Mary brought him up with this knowledge; surely as his brother, Jesus would have been brought up in this same custom.

If these texts are to be believed, we must ask: where did we stray? If Christ plainly taught these things according to so many sources, when did the rhetoric shift? It was well documented and known among many in the early Christian world that meat was not to be permitted. It wasn’t until the 4th century AD that Roman Emperor Constantine, who officially merged Christianity with Paganism to create a new state religion, gave the green light to meat consumption.[39] Since that time meat consumption has been generally accepted by most Christians.

If we accept that at least a portion of these texts are accurate, some may wonder, “why didn’t Joseph Smith make these changes in his translation of the Bible?” We can’t know for certain, but it appears that this was a principle Joseph was working to *restore*. The Apostle Peter taught of a restitution of all things, and this was merely a portion of what needed to be restored.[40] For instance, the Lord revealed to Joseph key changes to Genesis 9 that stipulated animals were only to be eaten to save life.[41] Joseph also received the revelation in Doctrine and Covenants 89 that essentially restored the diet given to Noah and confirmed Biblical teachings about intoxicating wine. Not only did the Prophet receive this instruction from the Lord, but he also taught the principles repeatedly to the Saints. Accepting all of this would lead us to believe that perhaps there are still things amiss in our KJV Bible about Christ and His use of fish–things that Joseph would have

---

[37] Eusebius, *Ecclesiastical History*, vol. 2, 23:5, translated by Arthur McGiffert.
[38] Howard Williams, *The Ethics of Diet*, (London, 1883), p. 56.
[39] See Steven Rosen, Food for the Spirit: Vegetarianism and the World Religions, (New York: Bala Books 1987).
[40] Acts 3:21.
[41] JST Genesis 9:10-11.

corrected had he been able to continue his work of translation on the Bible as he was planning before he was killed.

Regardless, we don't know for certain the veracity of these things. Did Christ really not partake of intoxicating wine and animal flesh? It's possible. However, we *do* know the things that were revealed to the Prophet Joseph Smith. It is hard to imagine that the Lord would not abide principles He would reveal to His prophet and expect His Saints to live. We can confidently assert that because Christ lived a sinless life, He took care of His mortal body by not defiling it with things He would later reveal to Joseph were harmful.

Acknowledgments

We have been so blessed to have the support of many friends and family members in our efforts to make this book a reality. First and foremost we would like to give a special thanks to Troy and Valerie Gundersen, Jordan's parents. They have been with us through every step of our journey and listened to all of our ideas—good and bad—without criticizing or dismissing. We could not have done this without them.

We also wouldn't have been able to do this without those who helped in the editing process by providing feedback and challenging some of our arguments. We would like to thank Cameron Bronson, Madeline Buhman, Jennifer Stinson, Threesa Cummings, Nicole Reeder, and Judy Shepherd.

Perhaps the most important part of making this book a reality was our launch team. The feedback they provided throughout the process was absolutely crucial from helping to name the book to promoting it on launch day. We would like to express our sincere thanks to Janelle Dunn, Alicia Spence, Matthew and Eliza Johnson, Pamela and Tyler Croall, Erica Rivera, Mariana and Jordan Keele, Lynette Keele, Abbey Hunziker, Cassidy Riddle, Callie Holbert, Becki Connolly, Timothy Steele, Alisa Eggiman, Jenny Colvin, Amanda Wyss, and Hannah Near.

We would also like to extend our gratitude to David and Jesse Christopher who were able to coordinate and help write the forward for the book on such short notice during a very busy time.

About the Authors

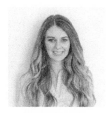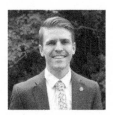

Cassidy and Jordan Gundersen met at and graduated from Brigham Young University. They are parents to two beautiful children. Together they own Spiro Health and Wellness, a company that they built to help people reverse chronic health conditions with diet. Their other hobbies include reading, hiking, Church history, and creating music.

Cassidy holds a Bachelor's degree in political science as well as a Master's degree in health and nutrition. She is also a nutritionist, health coach, and nutrition PhD candidate. She has educated audiences around the world about nutrition and health and has been featured at the United Nations, Eat Healthy Summit, Plant Based Utah, KSL, Well and Good Magazine, and Living Scriptures. If you would like to contact Cassidy, you can reach her at Cassidy@wordofwisdombook.com.

Jordan graduated from BYU with a Bachelor's degree in political science. If you ask him, his true passion is freedom—on a personal level and at a societal level—and blogs about it frequently. A number of years ago he started the Self Governance Project to help restore the ideas of personal responsibility and freedom. Before launching Spiro Health & Wellness, he was a business development manager managing a multi-million dollar portfolio for BestCompany.com. If you would like to contact Jordan, he can be reached at Jordan@wordofwisdombook.com.

Made in the USA
Las Vegas, NV
01 March 2022